GROW YOUR EYE CARE PRACTICE

High-Impact Pearls From
the Marketing Experts

GROW YOUR EYE CARE PRACTICE

High-Impact Pearls From the Marketing Experts

Editor

Ming Wang, MD, PhD
CEO, Aier-USA
Clinical Professor
Meharry Medical College
Director
Wang Vision Cataract & LASIK Center—An Aier-USA Eye Center
Co-Founder
The Common Ground Network
Nashville, Tennessee

Associate Editors

Shareef Mahdavi, BA, CEEE
President
SM2 Strategic
Pleasanton, California

Michael Malley, BA
Founder and President
CRM Group Marketing
Houston and Boerne, Texas

Tracy Schroeder Swartz, OD, MS, FAAO, Dipl ABO
Consultive Optometrist
The Laser Eye Center
Huntsville, Alabama

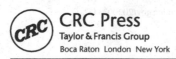

CRC Press
Taylor & Francis Group
Boca Raton London New York

CRC Press is an imprint of the
Taylor & Francis Group, an **informa** business

Cover Artist: Christine Seabo

First published 2021 by SLACK Incorporated

Published 2024 by CRC Press
2385 NW Executive Center Drive, Suite 320, Boca Raton FL 33431

and by CRC Press
4 Park Square, Milton Park, Abingdon, Oxon, OX14 4RN

CRC Press is an imprint of Taylor & Francis Group, LLC

© 2021 Taylor & Francis Group, LLC

Library of Congress Cataloging-in-Publication Data
Names: Wang, Ming X., 1960- editor. | Mahdavi, Shareef, editor. | Malley,
   Michael (Founder/president at Centre for Refractive Marketing), editor.
   | Swartz, Tracy Schroeder, editor.
Title: Grow your eye care practice : high-impact pearls from the marketing
   experts / edited by Ming Wang ; associate editors, Shareef Mahdavi,
   Michael Malley, Tracy Schroeder Swartz.
Description: Thorofare, NJ : SLACK Incorporated, [2021] | Includes
   bibliographical references and index.
Identifiers: LCCN 2020033452 (print) | ISBN 9781630917296 (paperback)

Subjects: MESH: Practice Management | Optometry--organization &
   administration | Ophthalmology--organization & administration |
   Marketing of Health Services
Classification: LCC RE72 (print) | NLM WW 704 | DDC
   617.70068--dc23
LC record available at https://lccn.loc.gov/2020033452

ISBN: 9781630917296 (pbk)
ISBN: 9781003524410 (ebk)

DOI: 10.1201/9781003524410

DEDICATION

To our families, patients, and colleagues.

CONTENTS

ACKNOWLEDGMENTS FROM THE EDITOR

I would like to express my sincere appreciation and gratitude toward the associate editors: Dr. Tracy Schroeder Swartz, for her hard work and dedication, and Mr. Shareef Mahdavi and Mr. Michael Malley, for their work in assisting Tracy. I would like to thank the team at SLACK Incorporated, with special thanks to Tony Schiavo.

I would like to also thank all the staff members of Wang Vision Cataract and LASIK Center—An Aier-USA Eye Center: Drs. Joshua Frenkel, Sarah Connolly, Nathan Rock, Marianne Johnson, Li Jiang, and Heather Brown; Clare Conway; Cameron Daniels; Suzanne Gentry; Alana Grimaud; Scott Haugen; Chloe Jenkins; Anle Ji; Baileh Kell; Amanda Knight; Haley Marcum; Ana Martinez; Shannon McClung; Eric Nesler; Beth Nielson; Ashley Patty; Kayla Sinyard; Clare Stolberg; Leona Walthorn; James Wright; and the entire Eye Surgery Center of Middle Tennessee team.

I have had the good fortune to have had the chance to learn from some great teachers over my professional career, including my laser spectroscopy PhD thesis advisor, Professor John Weiner; my MD (magna cum laude) thesis adviser and *Nature* paper coauthor, Professor George Church at Harvard Medical School and Massachusetts Institute of Technology; my ophthalmology residency advisors, Professors Larry Donoso and the late William Tasman at Wills Eye Hospital; my cornea and refractive surgery fellowship mentors, Professors Richard Forster, Scheffer Tseng, Eduardo Alfonso, Carol Karp, William Culbertson, and Lori Ventura at Bascom Palmer Eye Institute; my Vanderbilt University colleagues, the late Professors Dennis O'Day, James Elliott, and Donald Gass; and my colleagues at the Meharry Medical College.

I would like to thank my national and international colleagues as well, including Professors Arun C. Gulani, Jay Basal, Ilan Cohen, David Chang, Ron Krueger, Aleksandar Stonjavic, Guiseppe D'lppolito, Francis Muier, Steve Klyce, Marguerite McDonald, Dan Durrie, Steve Slade, George Waring, Terry Kim, Karl Stonecipher, Brian Boxer-Wachler, Terrence O'Brien, Jay Pepose, Guy Kezirian, Noel Alpins, Thomas Johns, Jack Holladay, Richard Lindstrom, Arlene Howard, Li Li, Bang Chen, Elaine Zhang, Chloe Chen, Jibo Zhou, Baosung Liu, Michael Zhou, Xiao-bing Wang, Zhi-yu Du, Qin-mei Wang, Jin-hai Huang, Li Zhen, David Liu, Jin-feng Chai, David Dai, Zu-guo Liu, Jun-wen Zen, David Fischer, Heather Ebert, David Dunham, John Mickner, Tony Ashley, Tony Roberts, Max Li, Dave and Jan Dalton, Jim and July Hiatt, Richard and Christine Nelson, Mike Fair, Charles Grummon, Jerry Moll, Carlos Enrique, Chenhua Yang, Kenny Markanich, Kip Dotson, and Kane Harrison.

Often one learns as much from fellows who he trains, and I have been fortunate to have a great group of doctors who have been my fellows over the years, including Drs. Shin Kang, Ilan Cohen, Uyen Tran, Walid Haddad, Mouhab Aljaheh, Ke-ming Yu, Yang-zi Jiang, Ray-Ann Lin, Lav Panchal, Lisa Marten, Lance Kugler, Michael George, Meagan Celmer, Marc Moore, Yang Yang, Ruibo Yang, Li Jiang, and Jibo Zhou. I have learned a great deal also from our optometry residents over the years, including Drs. Helen Boerman, David Coward, Shawna Hill, Tracy Winton, Dora Sztipanovits, Kevin Jackson, Ryan Vida, Bryce Brown, and Sarah Connolly.

Finally, I want to thank my family for their unfailing support and love: my wife, Anle Ji; my late father, Dr. Zhen-sheng Wang; my mother, Dr. Alian Xu; my brother, Dr. Ming-yu Wang; my son, Dennis Wang; my godmother, June Rudolph; and my godfather, Misha Bartnovsky.

—*Ming Wang, MD, PhD*

ACKNOWLEDGMENTS FROM THE ASSOCIATE EDITORS

Three key resources helped inform my contribution to this book. First are the many doctors I have had the privilege of working with over the years in my quest to help them be better in the their chosen profession. Next are Joe Pine and Jim Gilmore, coauthors of *The Experience Economy*, a book that forever changed the way I viewed the marketplace. And finally, our Creator, who has helped shape me in so many ways.

—*Shareef Mahdavi, BA, CEEE*

Special thanks to the hundreds of pioneering ophthalmic surgeons who have helped shape my passion, creative direction, and respect for ophthalmology during the past 30 years. Their inspiration and the endless support of my wife and business partner, Kandi, serve as quiet reinforcement that my efforts to properly market the benefits of our incredible industry have not gone unnoticed. Additional thanks to my 3 sons, Cole, Reid, and Will Malley, who make me the proudest father and coauthor on the planet.

—*Michael Malley, BA*

Thank you to my family, for supporting my endeavors, and Ming, for each and every opportunity he has given me. I am so thankful to all the doctors, professors, technicians, and professionals that helped shape me professionally and personally to allow me to be the person I am today. I am better for it.

—*Tracy Schroeder Swartz, OD, MS, FAAO, Dipl ABO*

About the Editor

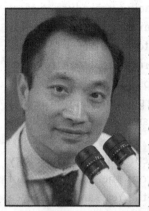

Ming Wang, MD, PhD is the CEO of Aier-USA, Director of Wang Vision Cataract & LASIK Center— An Aier-USA Eye Center, and clinical professor at Meharry Medical College, Nashville, Tennessee.

Growing up in China during the tumultuous Cultural Revolution, Dr. Wang played the Chinese violin er-hu and learned to dance in order to escape deportation and a life sentence of hard labor and poverty, a devastating fate that fell upon millions of youth. He came to the United States in 1982 with $50, a Chinese-English dictionary, and a big American dream in his heart. Dr. Wang graduated from Harvard Medical School and Massachusetts Institute of Technology (MD, magna cum laude) in Boston, Massachusetts; holds a doctorate degree in laser spectroscopy; and completed his residency in ophthalmology at Wills Eye Hospital in Philadelphia, Pennsylvania, and his corneal and refractive surgery fellowship at Bascom Palmer Eye Institute in Miami, Florida.

A former panel consultant to the US Food and Drug Administration Ophthalmic Device Panel and a founding director of Vanderbilt Laser Sight Center, Dr. Wang has published more than 120 scientific papers including a paper in the world-renowned journal *Nature* and numerous book chapters. He also has edited 9 ophthalmic textbooks including *Corneal Dystrophies and Degenerations: A Molecular Genetics Approach* and the following books published by SLACK Incorporated: *Corneal Topography in the Wavefront Era: A Guide for Clinical Application; Irregular Astigmatism: Diagnosis and Treatment; Keratoconus and Keratoectasia: Prevention, Diagnosis, and Treatment; Corneal Topography: A Guide for Clinical Application in the Wavefront Era, Second Edition; Atlas and Clinical Reference Guide for Corneal Topography; Refractive Lens Exchange: A Surgical Treatment for Presbyopia; Surgical Correction of Presbyopia: The Fifth Wave;* and *Grow Your Eye Care Practice: High-Impact Pearls From the Marketing Experts.*

Dr. Wang holds several US patents for his inventions of new biotechnologies to restore sight, including an amniotic membrane contact lens, an adaptive infrared retinoscopic device for detecting ocular aberrations, and a digital eye bank for virtual clinical trials. His invention of an amniotic membrane contact lens (for which he has obtained 2 US patents) has been used by more than 10,000 surgeons in the United States and worldwide in treating ocular surface diseases to restore sight. Dr. Wang is an investigator in the US Food and Drug Administration clinical trial of a sclera-spacing procedure to treat age-related loss of near vision (presbyopia) and ultraviolet cross-linking for the treatment of keratoconus. He introduced the femtosecond laser to China and performed China's first bladeless all-laser LASIK procedure using this laser in 2005. He also performed the world's first femtosecond laser–assisted artificial cornea implantation (Alphacor [Coopervision Surgical Inc]), and the first Intacs procedure in the United States using a new version of Intacs (Addition Technology, Inc) for advanced keratoconus.

Dr. Wang was a recipient of the American Academy of Ophthalmology Honor Award, the Lifetime Achievement Award from the Association of Chinese American Physicians, Kiwanis Nashvillian of the Year, and a Trevecca University honorary doctorate degree.

Dr. Wang is the CEO of Aier-USA, the US expansion of Aier Eye Hospital, the world's largest eye group with more than 500 locations in 3 of the 5 continents; the founding president of the Tennessee Chinese Chamber of Commerce; and cofounder of the Tennessee Immigrant and Minority Group. He founded a 501(c)(3) nonprofit organization named Wang Foundation for Christian Outreach to China.

Dr. Wang introduced many state-of-the-art technologies to the state including small incision lenticule extraction (SMILE), toric implantable contact lens, bladeless all-laser LASIK, laser refractive lens exchange for the treatment of presbyopia and laser refractive cataract surgery, Intacs and cross-linking for keratoconus, and an amniotic membrane contact lens. He runs a busy international referral clinic for post-LASIK and post–cataract surgery complications. Dr. Wang has performed more than 55,000 procedures (including on more than 4000 doctors), and the Wang Vision Cataract & LASIK Center— An Aier-USA Eye Center is currently the only center in the state that offers 3-dimensional (3D) SMILE and 3D LASIK (18 years or older), 3D implantable contact lens (21 years or older), 3D forever young lens (45 years or older), and 3D laser cataract surgery (60 years or older). He founded another 501(c)(3) nonprofit charity, the Wang Foundation for Sight Restoration, which has also helped patients from more than 40 states in the United States and 55 countries worldwide, with all sight restoration surgeries performed free of charge.

Dr. Wang is a champion amateur ballroom dancer and a former finalist in the world ballroom dance championships in the Open Pro-Am International 10 dance. He plays the er-hu and accompanied country music legend Dolly

Parton on her CD *Those Were the Days*. Dr. Wang organized an annual classical ballroom dance sight charity event, the EyeBall, and has drawn attendees from all over the United States and around the world.

The proceeds of Dr. Wang's autobiography, *From Darkness to Sight*, are donated to the 501(c)(3) nonprofit organization, the Wang Foundation for Sight Restoration, which is dedicated to helping blind orphan children from around the world. The book is being made into a full-length major motion picture.

ABOUT THE ASSOCIATE EDITORS

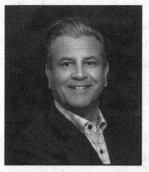

Shareef Mahdavi, BA, CEEE has worked with ophthalmologists since 1987 and held key sales and marketing leadership roles in the industry until starting his own advisory firm SM2 Strategic in 2001. Over the years, Mr. Mahdavi has advised thousands of doctors as well as dozens of companies on device launches, with a specific focus on the self-pay elective segment of health care. He has researched, written, and lectured extensively on the patient experience in refractive surgery; his work has been recognized by *The Experience Economy* coauthors Joseph Pine and Jim Gilmore for bringing customer experience principles to the refractive community. His work continues to expand into leveraging technology for better financial performance and improved operating efficiency in modern medical practice.

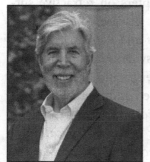

Michael Malley, BA is a former journalist who found his "content calling" in ophthalmology in 1988 when he founded CRM Group Marketing in Houston, Texas. Today, he is an annual lecturer at both the American Society of Cataract and Refractive Surgery in the United States and the European Society of Cataract & Refractive Surgeons in Europe and specializes in creative strategies that increase cataract and refractive surgical volume and enhance revenue streams. He consults with industry as well as many of the world's leading private ophthalmology practices and was so determined to better understand the frontline of ophthalmic marketing that he built and located his private consulting firm between a dedicated ophthalmic ambulatory surgery center and a comprehensive eye center.

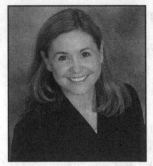

Tracy Schroeder Swartz, OD, MS, FAAO, Dipl ABO currently practices optometry specializing in anterior segment disease at the Laser Eye Center in Huntsville, Alabama. After completing her doctorate at Indiana University (Bloomington, Indiana), she pursued a master's degree in physiological optics while a clinical professor at the Indiana University School of Optometry. After completion of her master's degree, she relocated to Metro DC, where she specialized in refractive and corneal surgery and earned her fellowship in the American Academy of Optometry. She later joined Wang Vision Cataract & LASIK Center—An Aier-USA Eye Center in Nashville, Tennessee. Here, she served as Director of Clinical Operations, Residency Director for the Optometric Residency Program, and adjunct faculty to Indiana University School of Optometry. While there, she edited 2 textbooks with Ming Wang, MD, PhD: *Corneal Topography in the Wavefront Era: A Guide for Clinical Application* and *Irregular Astigmatism: Diagnosis and Treatment*, both published by SLACK Incorporated. She has authored numerous book chapters on refractive surgery, topography, aberrometry, and anterior segment disease. She served as coeditor for the literature review column for *Cataract and Refractive Surgery Today* from 2003 to 2008. She left Nashville for Huntsville, Alabama, in 2008 where she became the Center Director for VisionAmerica and became a diplomat of the American Board of Optometry. She edited additional books including *Keratoconus and Keratoectasia: Prevention, Diagnosis, and Treatment*; *Cornea Handbook*; *Corneal Topography: A Guide for Clinical Application in the Wavefront Era, Second Edition*; and *Surgical Correction of Presbyopia: The Fifth Wave*. She is President of the Optometric Cornea, Cataract and Refractive Society and served as the Education Chair for the organization for 10 years. She currently writes blogs for *Optometry Times* and https://odsonfb.com/ and consults for the industry.

CONTRIBUTING AUTHORS

Joshua Frenkel, MD, MPH (Chapter 17)
Anterior Segment Surgeon
Wang Vision Cataract & LASIK Center—An Aier-USA Eye Center
Nashville, Tennessee

Robbie W. Grayson III, BA (Chapters 4 and 17)
Stone Table School
Traitmarker
Traitmarker Books
Franklin, Tennessee

Arun C. Gulani, MD, MS (Chapter 17)
Founding Director and Chief Surgeon
Gulani Vision Institute
Global CEO
Gulani Vision Surgery Suites
Jacksonville, Florida
Externship Proctor
Midwestern University
Chicago, Illinois
Fellowship Faculty
Universitas Miguel Hernandez
Alicante, Spain
Faculty
International Researchers F1000Prime
London, United Kingdom

Kane Harrison (Chapters 8 and 16)
Founder and CEO
Vision Care Connect
Nashville, Tennessee

James E. Looper Jr, JD (Chapters 14 and 15)
Shareholder
Hall Booth Smitth, PC (National High Exposure Medical Litigation Group)
Nashville, Tennessee

Catherine Maley, MBA (Chapter 7)
Sausalito, California

John Mickner, BA (Chapters 10, 12, and 17)
COO
The Tennessee Immigrant and Minority Business Group
COO
The Tennessee American-Chinese Chamber of Commerce
Nashville, Tennessee

Karl Stonecipher, MD (Foreword)
Clinical Associate Professor of Ophthalmology
University of North Carolina
Chapel Hill, North Carolina
Medical Director
The Laser Center Greensboro
Greensboro, North Carolina

Michael Weiss, BS, MBA (Chapters 11 and 17)
CEO and Co-Founder
MedForward, Inc
Nashville, Tennessee

Jeremy Westby (Chapter 9)
President and CEO
2911 Enterprises, Inc
Nashville, Tennessee

PREFACE

Marketing for eye care providers has become one of the most important aspects of the eye care business today. Historically, the main challenge to a business was internal—how to make a product. Today, however, it is an external challenge—how to sell a product. The inversion of medical business dynamics, particularly related to elective procedures, is the result of an inversion of the supply and demand ratio. In the past, there were fewer eye doctors, and demand far exceeded supply. There was no need for marketing because the patients were abundant. Now, however, there are more eye care providers competing for patients who are often directed by their insurance plans. The need to attract patients has become the bottleneck of practice growth and has therefore also become the most important aspect of our business.

There is an unmet need to provide adequate education for eye care providers related to basic and practical marketing strategies. These are not topics that are discussed in medical or optometry schools or during residencies and fellowships. Most eye care providers are not successful with marketing due to the lack of education in this crucial area of business management.

Many of the most successful optometrists and ophthalmic (particularly refractive) surgeons were not only early adopters of new technologies and procedures, but they were also expert marketers.

To meet this critically important need, we have created this important and timely textbook, *Grow Your Eye Care Practice: High-Impact Pearls From the Marketing Experts*. Aggregating the teachings and experience in ophthalmic marketing from some of the leading practitioners internationally, this book is the first of its kind to provide a comprehensive education about the fundamentals of ophthalmic marketing. It offers practical tools to help eye care providers improve the most important aspect of today's practices.

The book first provides an overview of the history of ophthalmic marketing and points out why in the 21st century we need marketing more than ever before if we are to provide the highest quality in eye care. Specifically, a historical perspective is provided regarding LASIK vs presbyopic treatment marketing, and the commoditization of eye care is demonstrated by what happened with LASIK.

Next, we describe the basic strategies in ophthalmic marketing, including areas of classical marketing such as differentiation, market research, segmentation, targeting, and positioning. It explains why marketing includes more than just advertising; it should encompass the whole patient experience. It leads the reader to reconsider what their product really is—surgery, technology, or a service and patient experience? Branding vs call for action is discussed, and different strategies that one should employ are explored. Although word-of-mouth marketing is always the best, how to increase word-of-mouth referrals remains a big challenge, so we have devoted a chapter to this issue. The alignment of your marketing plan and your sales strategy is also discussed.

There has been a revolutionary increase in the development of tools that are available for marketing. Although traditional media such as radio, television, and print are still important and offer unique advantages, marketing via social media has taken over the world. Many eye care providers have been slow in adopting this change of landscape in marketing and are ill prepared to embrace social media technologies. In a section of the book, we describe all major social media marketing technologies and the best strategies to properly use them. We talk about websites, search engine optimization, and how to provide patients with efficient and effective online consultations. Topics include seminars, seasonal and topic-driven marketing, and other creative strategies.

In the next section, we discuss the ethics and laws that govern medical marketing. The health care industry is fundamentally different than other industries. As such, there are specific laws enacted that govern medical marketing, as well as various ethical issues.

The book concludes by describing some of the upcoming and disruptive technologies for marketing and the future directions of ophthalmic marketing.

Marketing is one of the most important aspects of our eye care practices today. We believe this textbook will be an indispensable desktop reference for eye care providers who desire to improve their marketing skills and grow their practices.

—*Ming Wang, MD, PhD*

FOREWORD

Quality is much better than quantity. One home run is much better than two doubles.

—Steve Jobs

Since antiquity, marketing has always been a part of everyday life. The Romans marketed anything from alcohol to bread to the most famous fish sauce, or garum.[1-4] Companies have risen and fallen based on clever market plans, and if you take a second to think about it, you will find jingles, favorite commercials, and past advertisements stuck in your head. So, what makes good marketing is a hot topic debated across board rooms and behind closed doors. The thought of "throwing money at it and see what sticks" no longer applies. Most businesses that are successful today spend a lot of energy on the following question: How do we reach the next customer?

Martin Luther King did not say "I have a mission statement."[5]
People don't buy what you do, they buy why you do it.[5]

—Simon Sinek

In Simon Sinek's famous speech "Start With Why," he notes the following:

There are people who walk around with Harley-Davidson tattoos on their bodies. That's insane. They've tattooed a corporate logo on their skin. Some of them don't even own the product! Why would rational people tattoo a corporate logo on their bodies? The reason is simple. After years of Harley being crystal clear about what they believe, after years of being disciplined about a set of values and guiding principles and after years of being doggedly consistent about everything they say and do, their logo has become a symbol.[5]

Last I checked, not one of my patients has "LASIK" or "Dr. Stonecipher ROCKS" tattooed on their body. How can we identify what makes a brand a brand or a logo a logo or a company a company? That is the ultimate answer to success. Is it luck? Is it skill? Is it talent? I would venture to guess it is a bit of all of that, but one thing we do know is that successful marketing is a team approach. It goes back to the lyrics "We get by with a little help from our friends." Paul McCartney and John Lennon wrote it with Ringo Starr singing the lyrics, and, of course, George Harrison played rhythm guitar, but there was also a producer—George Martin; it was recorded on the EMI label.

Social media is a contact sport.

—Margaret Molloy

I have had the opportunity to write with, work with, and know the editor, Dr. Ming Wang, and the associate editors, Shareef Mahdavi, Michael Malley, and Dr. Tracy Schroeder Swartz, for more than 20 years. The stellar lineup of this editorial board is without question more than "getting by with a little help from our friends." The lineup of authors contributing to this compendium of work are individuals who have "practiced what they have preached" into success stories year after year in up and down markets.

Marketing is really just about sharing your passion.

—Michael Hyatt

Marketing means different things to different people and practices. Marketing can be reference based, newsprint, television, radio, social media, internet, or just plain word of mouth. Practices, companies, and businesses have spent literally millions of dollars trying to brand a model, idea, technology, technique, or the surgeon or surgeons themselves. Patients and, for a better perspective, customers expect what they pay for in this market to change not only something physically but also something personally. They expect not only to walk away with what they purchased but also to enjoy the experience along the way. In today's world, the experience is what creates referrals and branding. The customer wants to know that you care about them and that the quality of what you provide is without question. I always like to finish a conversation with a surgical patient with the statement, "If you were one of my family members or me, this is exactly what I would be doing in this particular circumstance."

"Build it, and they will come" only works in the movies. Social media is a "build it, nurture it, engage them, and they may come and stay."

—Seth Godin

Mistakes in marketing are commonplace. It is how we learn from those mistakes that make us grow. Intention may be noble, but it may be bad timing, bad messaging, or the wrong outlet for that technology or group of individuals you are trying to reach. Tips from professionals like the authors of these chapters are priceless and may allow you to avoid the common phrase "experience means you have done it wrong before." The last thing you want to do is waste time or effort and, most importantly, limited resources when marketing.

People shop and learn in a whole new way compared to just a few years ago, so marketers need to adapt or risk extinction.

—Brian Halligan

One statistic that always has fascinated me is that out of 100 restaurants in New York City that open, only 10 will remain after a year (restaurant owner, New York City, personal communication). That gives new meaning to the "New York minute." Medicine has the success of attracting patients out of necessity but that does not mean choice does not exist. Of course, there are markets in which the "one-man band" exists, but in this day that is a rare occurrence. Competition is the normal, not the exception.

Advertising brings in customers, but word of mouth brings in the best customers.

—Jonah Berger

Reputation takes years to cultivate but moments to lose. Your last marketing campaign only works if you provide consistent quality of service. I am constantly reminding my staff that the customer is always right no matter how wrong he or she may be. The chapters of this book outline traditional and not-so-traditional methods of marketing. They illustrate ways to spend money and ways to save money on social media or word-of-mouth campaigns. Most importantly, they discuss the legal and ethical sides to marketing and that in itself could prove to be one of the best lessons learned from this textbook.

Our jobs as marketers are to understand how the customer wants to buy and help them to do so.

—Bryan Eisenberg

Each of the editors and contributing authors to this textbook has encountered real-world consumers. They are not counting widgets in some ivory tower. That concept is the beauty of this collaboration. These individuals deal with day-to-day marketing issues in the day-to-day world and have done it over the course of time. What those of us who have been around for a while have come to understand is that marketing is not static. It is a dynamic endeavor changing from day to day, city to city, and practice to practice.

Give them quality. That is the best kind of advertising.

—Milton Hershey

Most textbooks become reference sources that sit on the shelf and are only read in bits and pieces. This textbook will be one you will want to read from cover to cover like the latest suspense thriller novel. Not only is it filled with expertise beyond belief, but it also will save you thousands of dollars in opinions that are summed up in its pages. The chapters cover marketing from A to Z and provide you with multiple ideas to instill in your practice, whether it be small or large. The suggestions in this book should allow you to make decisions that will influence your practice and provide you with the opportunity to grow whatever model you chose. Success is not achieved by sitting on the sidelines, and this reference source will not only get you in the game, but it will also help excel you across the goal line.

—*Karl Stonecipher, MD*

References

1.   Maran J, Stockhammer PW, eds. *Materiality and Social Practice: Transformative Capacities of Intercultural Encounter.* Oxbow; 2012.
2.   Demirdjian ZS. Rise and fall of marketing in Mesopotamia: a conundrum in the cradle of civilization. In: Neilson L, ed. *The Future of Marketing's Past: Proceedings of the 12th Annual Conference on Historical Analysis and Research in Marketing.* Association for Analysis and Research in Marketing; 2005:102-115.
3.   Dobbins JJ, Foss PW. *The World of Pompeii.* Routledge; 2008:330.
4.   Curtis RI. A personalized floor mosaic from Pompeii. *Am J Archaeol.* 1984;88(4):557-566. doi:10.2307/504744
5.   Sinek S. *Start With Why: How Great Leaders Inspire Everyone to Take Action.* Penguin Group; 2009.

Section I

History of Ophthalmic Marketing
and Perspectives

1

The History of Ophthalmic Marketing

Michael Malley, BA

The genesis of ophthalmic marketing has its beginnings more than 4000 years ago near Cairo, Egypt. Medical folklore tells of a minimally trained "eye specialist" who convinced a blind Egyptian to allow him to take an instrument known as a *lancet* to manually push his clouded lens backward into the vitreous cavity and leave it there. Although hyperopic, the man's vision was brighter, allowing him to function as a productive member of society. That man went on to tell his neighbors how this procedure changed his life. Word-of-mouth ophthalmic marketing was born. This method of marketing became an effective refractive marketing technique.

Word-of-mouth marketing continued to grow when French surgeon-oculist Jacques Daviel reported to the French Academy of Surgery in 1752 that he had performed the first modern cataract surgery by making a corneal incision and removing a cataract. England continued the advancement of cataract surgery

Wang M, ed. *Grow Your Eye Care Practice:*
High-Impact Pearls From the Marketing Experts (pp 3-5).

in 1949 when Harold Ridley implanted the first intraocular lens addressing refractive error. Now, patients undergoing vision correction surgery share stories of visual restoration by mouth and social media.

The Federal Trade Commission (FTC) has regulated medical marketing since 1914. The Federal Trade Commission Act was passed then to empower the FTC to regulate unfair methods of competition in commerce, including deceptive ophthalmic advertising. In fact, companies advertising radial keratometry (RK) were sued by the FTC for false and misleading advertising. The outcome was the establishment of many ophthalmic marketing guidelines that are still in place.

As the prevalence of marketing procedures such as RK, astigmatic keratotomy, and anterior lamellar keratoplasty grew in the 1980s, professionals started to advertise cataract surgery. The 3 main affiliate television partners (ABC, CBS, and NBC) offered an opportunity for progressive surgeons to reach massive viewing audiences interested in vision correction. At the time, advertising by doctors was frowned upon, and some surgeons were ridiculed for doing so.

The leading edge of direct response marketing in the 1980s was radio. Prospective vision correction patients were targeted by selecting various formats of radio stations. RK marketing messaging in the 1980s focused on the benefit of seeing well at distance without the need for glasses or contact lenses. Patient testimonial campaigns and media interviews with surgeons talking about the new procedures were used.

In 1990, surgeons in Europe and Canada were replacing RK, astigmatic keratotomy, and anterior lamellar keratoplasty with excimer laser technology. The public fell in love with phototherapeutic keratectomy followed by LASIK. More laser refractive correction procedures were performed in the 1990s than any other decade. It was not until the late 1990s that websites were developed. Ophthalmic marketing in the 1990s continued to use mainly traditional media. LASIK centers started taking out full-page print ads and running paid 30-minute infomercials on major networks. According to MarketScope, consumer awareness of the term LASIK by men and women wearing either glasses or contacts peaked at over 90% in the 1990s.

The next decade brought ophthalmic websites, reputation management, online patient reviews, social media, retargeting, Google AdWords, search engine optimization, click-through rates, and cost per lead. Modern word-of-mouth marketing is called *influencer marketing*. It still involves happy patients talking about their procedure, but the audience is well outside traditional boundaries. Today's "friends" include "followers" and people who "like" and "share" ophthalmic stories on social media.

This has led to metrics marketing. Marketing budgets and surgical volume are based on data analytics. Marketing budgets are based on the amount of marketing dollars to create an impression and generate leads. Leads become office visits, and more office visits drive surgical volume. Professionals direct the right messaging with the right media to create the desired result.

Although word of mouth remains an important type of marketing, it has become far more complicated.

LASIK Versus Presbyopic Marketing

A Perspective

Michael Malley, BA

From my personal ophthalmic marketing perspective, the view could not get any better. Everyone will eventually become presbyopic and similarly develop cataracts. The general public surely does not enjoy the same favorable perspective as I do. For most of the readers of this text, these conditions represent a tremendous opportunity to restore clear vision to the largest segment of aging eyes in medical history. From a refractive surgeon's perspective, the view is excellent. People with presbyopia develop cataracts that need to be surgically removed. More people than ever will be visiting an eye care provider near them to have lens replacement surgery during the next decade. The question you need to ask yourself is "Will it be you?"

Here is more good news for refractive surgeons: Before people become presbyopic and develop cataracts, more than half of them will develop refractive error and require glasses or contact lenses. That makes for a sizable potential LASIK market. Unfortunately, the conversion to LASIK is a fraction of the conversion for cataract surgery.

Wang M, ed. *Grow Your Eye Care Practice:
High-Impact Pearls From the Marketing Experts* (pp 7-14).
© 2021 Taylor & Francis Group.

From a marketing perspective, the immediate discernible difference between presbyopia and LASIK is the penetration rate for LASIK. It remains under 10% for the 52% of people who are nearsighted, farsighted, and astigmatic. For reasons of either fear or financial concerns, 95% of the population prefers to remain in glasses or contacts vs LASIK, which is not good news for refractive surgeons.

With only 5% of the population choosing to have LASIK compared with over 90% of the population who at some point will undergo cataract surgery or refractive lens exchange (RLE), it is important that refractive surgeons not lose their financial focus. As the most successful and popular vision correction procedure ever developed, LASIK has been a tremendous procedure for patients and surgeons alike. However, for comprehensive refractive anterior segment surgeons, rarely will LASIK provide the same potential revenue stream, surgical volume, and extended patient satisfaction as cataract surgery.

If time management and profit margins are a concern, I would recommend focusing first on building and growing a cataract practice. Focus on building or maintaining your LASIK practice with the remaining time and resources. I have seen too many practices invest a disproportionate percentage of their marketing budget to LASIK when it represents only a fraction of practice revenue compared with lens implant procedures and ambulatory surgery center revenue.

THE DAWN OF PRESBYOPIC MARKETING

There is one main difference between a LASIK patient and a presbyopic patient—the person with presbyopia has money. They are in the core earning stage of life and have the financial resources and purchasing power to afford nonessential medical procedures like laser-assisted cataract surgery or RLE. Access to more disposable income is possibly why the average person having LASIK today is in his or her mid-30s.

Another subtle difference between LASIK patients and patients with presbyopia is their spectacles. Prescription glasses are becoming more vogue and fashionable. LASIK patients do not have the same distaste for glasses as in the past. There is nothing fashionable about reading glasses. They are an instant identifier of aging.

Marketing surgical correction for presbyopia has never been much of a challenge and remains simple. You target the middle-aged population and tell them you have an exciting alternative that will help them see better and look younger without reading glasses. This simple yet effective primary message has worked well.

The problem with presbyopia marketing has not been the messaging or the media but rather that the numerous presbyopia-correcting procedures have failed. They failed to impress the public enough to elect to have them and failed to be a permanent and long-term solution for consistent near vision. Therefore, most practices have abandoned attempts to provide patients with a solution for temporarily correcting presbyopia.

Modern surgeons market laser lens replacement and RLE to permanently correct presbyopia. This can be highly effective for the right candidate with proper expectations using appropriate technology. Problems arise when doctors overpromise and underdeliver, creating a postoperative nightmare. Proceed with caution surgically as we discuss the "marketing holy grail" of refractive surgery.

A SLOWER-MOVING MARKETING TARGET

Unlike illusive younger millennials who are never far from a mobile device, tablet, or laptop and are constantly inundated with retargeting banners and social media messages, the middle-aged person with presbyopia is a more settled target audience with more predictable patterns. This is advantageous for marketers. People with presbyopia are more susceptible to advertising because they are less engaged and less inundated than millennials. They are busy at home, making them an easier target. This is especially true for traditional media like television or radio.

Eye care providers may think traditional media methods are old school, but there is a good reason why major cellular companies, mobile device manufacturers, major food chains, soft drink brands, and beer manufacturers continue to use traditional media. These methods work in getting a message delivered in a somewhat private setting like the home or car to a vast market audience. These are significant mass appeal media partners that can deliver the largest target audiences in your market. In contrast to the naysayers who have gone all in on digital, there is an absolute place for television and radio for presbyopia marketing.

Radio Advertising for Presbyopia

For radio, attract middle-aged people by focusing on "active listenership" stations offering news, traffic, weather, and sports. Although Pandora and SiriusXM radio are options for listening pleasure, most potential candidates who are fighting traffic going to and from work each day are still listening to local radio. A higher frequency of shorter commercials is better than longer, low frequency commercials, so buying 15-second traffic and weather sponsorships every half hour on the hour is better than 60-second commercials that air run of schedule. Run of schedule spots (ie, spots that are more affordable but the station can run them outside of your scheduled times) run at the station's discretion and are not recommended. Radio also works best when you have influencer marketing engaged with popular program hosts discussing visual freedom from reading glasses.

Television Advertising for Presbyopia

Follow the same approach for television. Live, upscale sporting events are best. Middle-aged audiences watch more of them live than recorded. Professional golf, tennis, and college football have more upper-income viewership, but their total viewing is lower than professional football, basketball, and baseball. The evening news at 10 or 11 PM also has strong active viewership by people who stay involved in their local community. Shorter 15-second TV commercials allow you to buy more frequency than 30-second commercials. Buying remnant inventory on cable stations can be a nice addition to a local affiliate TV buy (ABC, CBS, or NBC). During political seasons, focus on major cable news networks for each side of the political fence. People with presbyopia do not tend to have one party affiliation, so you will need to buy both.

Internet and Social Media Advertising for Presbyopia

An online search for presbyopia correction is a small fraction of the search volume compared with LASIK. This makes AdWords advertising with Google more affordable for presbyopia correction than LASIK, allowing practices to maintain a strong presence in an uncrowded field. Because the search volume is low, a more effective digital campaign would include Facebook and Instagram. As more millennials depart these platforms for Twitter, Snapchat, and others, people with presbyopia and cataract patients are growing on Facebook.

Paid banner ads showing people with presbyopia reading restaurant menus, recipes, text messages, and emails without reading glasses is a simple, effective strategy. Make reading glasses a part of every headline. Viewers make an immediate connection because they feel nothing positive about wearing reading glasses. Comments such as "Looking older than you feel in readers?" will get their attention.

CREATIVE PRESBYOPIC MESSAGING

Forget using the word *presbyopia* or *presbyopic* in your advertising unless you first explain it. Unlike the word LASIK that has over 95% brand awareness, the word presbyopia means nothing to the general public. What they understand the most are "reading glasses," "granny glasses," and "cheaters." They understand they have lost their ability to see up close. People with presbyopia also are not familiar with the word refractive and have shown a negative connotation with the word extraction, probably because it is associated with dentistry. Few people feel warm and fuzzy about a clear lens extraction, so change the terminology to either laser lens replacement or RLE. There is no negative association with refractive, so RLE is probably the best acronym to use.

Looking younger and seeing better are 2 attractive qualities of having a lens exchange procedure. The marketing message "Want to see BETTER and look YOUNGER?" is recommended. Another attraction for patients in their 50s and early 60s is that they will never need to undergo cataract surgery. They are intrigued by this message, but it needs a little explanation for patients to fully understand the concept.

THE COST BENEFIT OF PRESBYOPIA CORRECTION

It is not uncommon for practices to perform LASIK on patients well into their 50s and 60s. As long as patients understand their lack of near vision will continue even when monovision LASIK is performed, this method of LASIK has been shown to be successful for surgeons and welcomed by patients. If performed before cataract surgery, this can be expensive. Paying $4000 for LASIK when you are 50 years old and then $8000 for bilateral laser cataract surgery with multifocal lenses is a substantial financial pill to swallow.

A proven way to make presbyopic lens exchange affordable is to present patients with the following options: The patient could have LASIK for $4000, but refractive cataract surgery will be needed later for $6000. Having RLE for $8000 is more affordable in the long run, and the patient will never need cataract surgery. This discussion makes a permanent presbyopic procedure a more affordable option for patients who understand the long-term benefits.

LASIK Marketing

Before the corporate LASIK discounters got involved, LASIK was *not* a commodity. It was an advanced, proven, safe, and accurate vision correction procedure that was far superior to previous radial keratotomy and lamellar keratoplasty procedures. The public quickly embraced LASIK, and people were willing to pay the going rate for the procedure. LASIK marketing began in the 1990s, and most advertising was benefit based. You simply advertised the benefit of LASIK compared with the former bladed radial keratotomy and lamellar keratoplasty procedures. Outcomes were stable. There was no hyperopic shift. The word laser indicated precision, accuracy, and safety. LASIK brand awareness was over 90% by men and women with refractive error.

Unfortunately, in the midst of the most successful run in ophthalmic marketing history, corporate discounters turned LASIK into a commodity. No longer were marketing campaigns focused on the benefits of LASIK. They were all about price. This was misleading, confusing, and devastating for surgeons. Prospective patients cared less about technology and outcomes and more about fees, financing, and monthly payments. When the value of a $4000 bilateral laser procedure is suddenly offered for as little as $199 per eye, it drives down the overall value of the procedure. If only the public had known that no legitimate LASIK candidate ever received surgery for $199. It was a true "bait and switch."

This combined with the 9/11 attack in 2001 marked the beginning of the end of LASIK. As the national marketing spending on LASIK trended down after 9/11 so did surgical volume. By the economic crisis in 2008, the national LASIK volume was significantly reduced. The LASIK market has *never* recovered to the level enjoyed in the 1990s.

The current LASIK volume has been flat for years with little growth. Corporate discount LASIK centers who continue to generate patients by insinuating you can have LASIK for as little as $220 per eye are the only sector seeing growth. Effective ways to compete with value-brand LASIK corporate discounters are as follows:

- Offer seasonal savings ($500 to $1000).
- Offer a best LASIK price guarantee for your technology.
- Offer a 20/20 commitment for patients who qualify.

- Expose them with white papers ("Beware of Bait-n-Switch LASIK").
- Introduce new LASIK technology, such as iDesign 2.0 (Johnson & Johnson Vision) and Contoura Vision (Alcon).
- Reward prospects for coming in for LASIK consults.

METRICS MARKETING

As discussed earlier, metrics are helping transform LASIK marketing from an art to an actual science. Metrics are an excellent way to establish goals and benchmarks from year to year. All you need to know are your conversion factors on the following:

Total leads coming into the practice = online leads + phone calls + text messages + form completions

To accurately benchmark and set goals, track conversion percentages. Track what is happening to every lead and inquiry coming into the practice. If you only convert 3% to 4% of online leads to office visits, and you need 10 LASIK office visits per week to generate 20 eyes per week in surgery, you will need in excess of 200 leads per month to meet your goals. You then need to know how much it costs the practice to generate over 200 online leads.

If your conversion from phone calls is higher than online leads, which it should be, then determine what you need to spend to generate more calls. Determine what it costs to generate those calls and build it into your budget. Soon you will become more precise in predicting both your marketing spending and your surgical volume.

The same format applies to text message generation and form completions. Monitor the conversion and determine the marketing budget to perform the projected surgical volume. You also have to understand the rates of LASIK consultation no-shows, consultation cancellations, LASIK noncandidates, and LASIK conversion from a good candidate to surgery.

These numbers can be sobering because of the amount of money you are spending on LASIK compared with the volume of surgery you are performing. Your efforts may appear to be generating strong impressions, a high volume of leads, and a strong overall interest in your LASIK messaging. The best indicator is the amount of surgical volume. With metrics marketing, the easiest and most cost-effective way to reduce your marketing spending and increase your surgical volume is to increase conversion rates.

Although most LASIK patients love their vision after they have had it done, most patients do not have the foresight to see themselves post-LASIK. They focus on everything that happens in the pre-LASIK process. Always talk in post-LASIK terms. For instance, "I am excited for you to wake up the morning after your LASIK procedure and see the clock," or "Imagine taking care of your baby in the middle of the night without glasses." Higher conversions result when you encourage patients to see the benefits of LASIK before surgery. This increases the value of the procedure. The goal is to determine what patients are most passionate about and describe how much better that pursuit will be with freedom from glasses.

3

Commoditization
What Happened to LASIK?

Shareef Mahdavi, BA, CEEE

As an economic term, *commoditization* refers to a process in which a good or service becomes difficult to distinguish from other similar offerings over time. As a result, purchase decisions are made primarily on price because there is little besides prices to differentiate the offering.

THE GREAT PRICING EXPERIMENT OF 2000–2002

We are now approaching the 20th anniversary of the great pricing experiment in LASIK in which providers believed they could grow consumer demand for LASIK, and all forms of laser vision correction, by lowering the fee charged to the consumer. Beginning in late 1999, we saw the emergence of discount LASIK providers among several corporate chain groups and individual surgeon practices. Although LASIK fees had averaged above $2000 before this

Wang M, ed. *Grow Your Eye Care Practice:*
High-Impact Pearls From the Marketing Experts (pp 15-22).
© 2021 Taylor & Francis Group.

point, by midyear 2000, 1 in 10 refractive surgeons was offering LASIK below $1000 per eye, with many starting at under $500 per eye.

The situation was encouraged by the leading excimer manufacturer VISX (now Johnson & Johnson Vision), which in December 1999 lost a major legal battle against Nidek Inc. The International Trade Commission had determined that Nidek Inc was not infringing on patents held by VISX, and the verdict justified the per-procedure fees charged to owners of the laser. The response by Wall Street was immediate and ominous; the company's stock lost nearly 40% of its value overnight, and trading was temporarily halted on the NASDAQ exchange.

Several months later in February 2000, VISX lowered the per-procedure royalty fee from $250 to $110 per eye. The company positioned this as part of a "Strategic Growth Initiative," which was intended to spur market growth by lowering costs to providers in the channel of distribution between the laser manufacturer and the consumer. The manufacturer encouraged its customers to lower their fees to patients with the belief that this would translate to higher consumer demand for the procedure.

MARKET RESEARCH

There were no market data at the time to suggest that lower prices would stimulate greater demand among patients. On the contrary, independent consumer surveys conducted showed that price, specifically a low price offering, was not relevant to consumers, with only 8% saying price was significant in their decision making.[1]

Doctors and practices offering laser vision correction were seeking ways to better educate patients and help them overcome their fear of refractive procedures. The market had grown rapidly from the initial Food and Drug Administration approval in 1996, and prices had increased in tandem as shown in the early data points to the left of Figure 3-1.

What happened to the demand for LASIK? I authored a series of articles published from 2002 to 2005[2,3] in which this question was studied, analyzed, and reported, with data analysis on the relationship between average fees and overall demand in the United States for subsequent years. The clear conclusion from the data is that lowering the price failed to increase demand.

Although we cannot prove cause and effect, we can demonstrate a high correlation between the average fee charged for LASIK each year and the overall

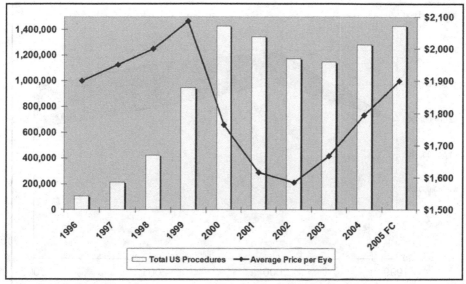

Figure 3-1. The price of vision correction procedures rose from initial US Food and Drug Administration approval in 1996, peaking in 1999, falling in 2000, and slowly rising. Procedures performed peaked in 2000, falling slightly as prices fell in 2002, and then steadily rose.

procedure volume the following year. Economists do this routinely, looking at the elasticity of demand relative to the price charged. Pricing theory suggests that the demand for a good or service is elastic if overall demand increases when unit pricing falls. Conversely, economists say that demand is inelastic if demand does not grow when pricing is lowered.

As a health care offering, LASIK clearly shows inelasticity of demand. Although demand suffered after the fall of prices, demand subsequently improved as pricing levels increased back toward their pre-experiment highs.

At the 2003 American Society of Cataract and Refractive Surgery meeting, I presented a paper[4] showing the harmful effect of commoditization of LASIK that was being attempted through the lowering of fees. The punch line to the talk is that over the 3-year period from 2000 to 2002, reduced prices led to nearly a $1.7 billion reduction of top-line revenue for the profession because the price for LASIK had decreased by $428 on average per eye during this 3-year period. Because fixed costs did not decrease, that meant that $1.7 billion of operating margin was eroded because of the discounting, which averaged $335,000 per refractive surgeon active at that time. You could hear a pin drop at the end of my talk, which was, incidentally, awarded Best Paper of Session (Figure 3-2).

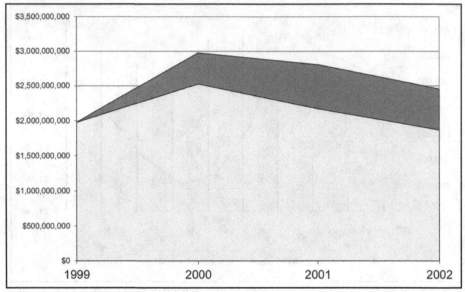

Figure 3-2. The cost of LASIK fell an average of $428 per eye from 2000 to 2002, resulting in a loss of $1.7 billion in profits cumulatively for all LASIK providers.

BUT LASIK IS DIFFERENT

Before that presentation, surgeons and industry pundits believed that LASIK volume had dropped because of outside events, such as the dot-com meltdown in early 2000, the economic recession that followed, and societal change caused by the events of September 11, 2001. These explanations seemed plausible but failed to account for the pricing behavior initiated by laser owners. To better understand what was causing the decline in volume, I began looking into other elective procedures to see what happened to them during this time period. Annual surveys of cosmetic procedures data[5] published by the American Society of Plastic Surgery contained pricing and procedure volume data for many procedures including breast augmentation.

Breast augmentation shares similarities to laser vision correction in that it is elective, is typically performed bilaterally with similar surgical fees, and is done on an outpatient basis with modest recovery and immediate results. With this in mind, I chose to analyze the available data on total US procedure volume and average surgeon fees, using it as a control group to compare with LASIK.

The result, as shown in Figure 3-3, was a startling contrast when comparing the 2 procedures each year. Unlike the "roller-coaster" pattern seen in LASIK,

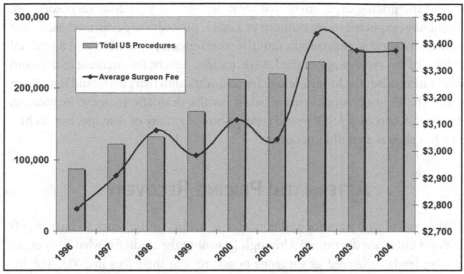

Figure 3-3. Unlike LASIK, breast augmentation increased in performed procedures as well as price during the same time period.

the relationship between price and volume for breast augmentation moved in the same direction. Overall, although prices went up by 21%, the overall procedure demand tripled. Indeed, plastic surgery was showing a similar inelasticity of demand but in the opposite direction. This pattern is also seen in the price/demand relationship for luxury goods and services where demand tends to increase as prices rise.

The breast augmentation category showed significant growth in demand as prices increased during the same period that LASIK showed declines in both demand and average fees. The data comparison deflated the argument that the drop in LASIK demand could be attributed mainly to external factors as described previously because both specialties were subject to the same influences. One plastic surgeon friend that reviewed the findings bluntly asked, "What's wrong with those ophthalmologists?" as he indicated how much his practice had grown because of the increasing availability of surgical and nonsurgical esthetic treatments (personal communication, oral).

Additional research into hearing aids showed a similar conclusion regarding inelasticity of demand. Numerous studies[6] published by Amyn Amlani, PhD, a professor of audiology, indicate that the demand for hearing aids does not increase when prices are lowered. This is part of a larger conclusion around elective health care—it is very difficult, if not impossible, to create demand simply by lowering the price.

Had the pricing experiment that took hold in the year 2000 succeeded, we would have expected to see millions of LASIK procedures performed each year with an increasing penetration into the nearsighted population and a gradual decline of the average age of the LASIK patient. Likely, the increase in demand would have offset the lower average fee and, although margins would have been lower, the industry would thrive based on the dramatic increase in volume. Had that occurred, LASIK would clearly show elasticity of demand, but, as history has shown, that did not occur.

AFTERMATH: PRICING RECOVERY

The goal of every author and educator is for his or her work to have an effect and influence the future. Although I cannot take credit for what happened, pricing levels recovered as surgeons began raising their fees in 2003. The introduction of the femtosecond laser and customized treatment provided new technology at a higher cost, which was passed on to consumers. Average fees, which had fallen below $1600 in 2002, rose and by 2007 had once again crossed the $2000 per eye mark. Not surprisingly, procedure volumes were moving back toward their peak, which had last been seen in 2000 when 1.4 million procedures were performed.

In late 2008, another recession began, which halted LASIK's recovery in its tracks. Volumes fell dramatically, dropping to approximately 650,000 eyes. Without question, the shift in the economy had created havoc for elective procedures, including LASIK and plastic surgery.

One interesting development ocurred in pricing. Average fees for LASIK remained steady and stable for more than a decade since the great recession of 2008. However, plastic surgeons lowered their fees in the subsequent years. During the same period, procedure volumes stayed flat or fell. Again, we make no assertion about cause and effect, which is much more difficult to prove. However, refractive surgeons are to be commended for not repeating the same mistake and learning from the failed attempt to commoditize LASIK through discount pricing.

More broadly, commoditization includes the reputation of the procedure as well as its pricing. LASIK's reputation has indeed suffered because too much emphasis has been put on the technology and too little on the impact on the life of the patient. The damage done in the early 2000s by low pricing has given way to the damage done by chronic negative publicity, including the recent suicide of a TV anchor after a small incision lenticule extraction procedure.[7] The fear induced by this information is significant and difficult to overcome in the short term because the alternative to laser vision correction is to continue wearing glasses, which poses no risk and no immediate cost.

Fear remains a factor that needs to be respected and managed effectively as part of the patient's overall experience in his or her decision-making process. Had fear no longer been an issue, it is feasible that LASIK procedures could have grown via lower pricing and exhibited elasticity of demand as described earlier.

PRICING STRATEGY

My hope with this historical review of pricing in laser vision correction is that surgeons will realize that they have control in how they set fees and what they offer for that price. My colleague, customer service expert John DiJulius,[8] has often said that businesses should think of their fees in terms of 2 categories: the basics, which is what everybody offers, and the customer service tax, which is the premium charged because your offering includes a high service component that is valued by the customer, as is the case in "boutique" practices. If you cannot justify the premium tax assessment in your offering, you have not earned the right to assess it according to DiJulius.

Harvard Business School Professor Frances Frei makes the same point, albeit a bit differently, in her book *Uncommon Service: How to Win by Putting Customers at the Core of Your Business*,[9] where she distinguishes between hygiene factors and motivating factors. *Hygiene factors* refer to any attribute of the business that is expected and does not serve to motivate the consumer. However, the lack of its presence will prevent repeat business. Think of the great food at the restaurant with the unkept washroom; you are likely not going back. A true motivating factor is one that is neither anticipated nor expected; it makes the consumer want to choose you over other providers. It is often unique and memorable.

Focus on identifying and incorporating true motivators if you want to be in a position to charge a premium. Always remember that today's motivator may become tomorrow's hygiene factor. One hotel chain's unique "heavenly bed"[10] has now been emulated by just about everybody in the hotel business and is no longer a special, differentiating feature.

CONCLUSION

Without question, when 2 offerings are viewed as similar with indistinguishable features and benefits, most consumers will choose the one with the lower cost. That is the definition of a commodity. Examine your own behavior when shopping on Amazon or at an auto dealership. For the exact same product, you will likely choose the one with the lower price.

With LASIK, the key is for surgeons to develop a highly distinguishable offering, one that cannot easily be compared with what is offered down the street. Differentiation, a key marketing element, should be the goal of every LASIK provider who wants to be viewed as unique, special, and worth whatever he or she charges in the mind of the consumer.

How one achieves meaningful differentiation is a matter of debate among marketing experts. My view on this subject will be addressed in another chapter in this book on customer experience.

REFERENCES

1. Mahdavi S. Retail pricing in refractive surgery, part III. *Cataract Refract Surg Today*. 2005;November:82-84.
2. Mahdavi S. Retail pricing in refractive surgery. *Cataract Refract Surg Today*. 2002;October:29-38.
3. Mahdavi S. Retail pricing in refractive surgery, part II. *Cataract Refract Surg Today*. 2003;June:39-42.
4. Mahdavi S. Retail pricing in refractive surgery. Paper presented at: American Society of Cataract and Refractive Surgery Annual Meeting; April 12, 2003; San Francisco, CA.
5. American Society of Plastic Surgeons. Plastic surgery statistics. Accessed August 3, 2020. https://www.plasticsurgery.org/news/plastic-surgery-statistics
6. Amlani A. Impact of elasticity of demand on price in the hearing aid market. *Audiology Online*. January 29, 2007. Accessed August 3, 2020. https://www.audiologyonline.com/articles/impact-elasticity-demand-on-price-955
7. Kindelan K, Messervia S. Family of meteorologist says she had eye surgery complications before suicide. ABC channel 15, Arizona. Accessed April 28, 2019. https://www.abc15.com/national/family-of-meteorologist-says-she-had-eye-surgery-complications-before-suicide
8. DiJulius J. *Secret Service: Hidden Systems That Deliver Unforgettable Customer Service*. AMACOM; 2003.
9. Frei F. *Uncommon Service: How to Win by Putting Customers at the Core of Your Business*. Harvard Business Review Press, Boston; 2012.
10. Westin Store. The heavenly bed. Accessed August 3, 2020. https://www.westinstore.com/category.aspx?The-Heavenly-Bed

Section II

Basic Marketing Strategies

4

Market Research and Segmentation, Targeting, and Positioning

Robbie W. Grayson III, BA

The health of any business rises and falls on how accurately it can answer the following questions:

- Who is my customer?
- Where is my customer?
- What does my customer need from me?
- How do I get my customer's attention?

Market research is an art, but it was first a science. Understanding the science gives one the ability to creatively cultivate the art of getting customers. In the United States, the history of market research has its origin in the early 20th century.

Daniel Starch (1883–1979) was the first American market researcher on the scene. It appears that he was the first to come up with a formal system for "getting into the customer's head."[1] In his book *Advertising: Its Principles, Practices,*

Wang M, ed. *Grow Your Eye Care Practice:*
High-Impact Pearls From the Marketing Experts (pp 25-33).
© 2021 Taylor & Francis Group.

and Techniques, Starch[1] explains how he merged psychology and advertising to create a market research strategy that involved door-to-door canvassing of neighborhoods.

AIDED RECALL

According to Starch, his process involved finding the subscribers of specific newspapers and magazines. That meant that he had to walk hundreds of miles and knock on hundreds of doors to find enough subscribers to interview. Once he found a consenting subscriber, he would guide him or her through a series of ads in the newspaper or magazine of relevance, occasionally stopping to ask specific questions about the ads. Based on the subscriber's answers, he would give a grade. Once compiled, those grades gave him information about subscriber behavior.

Actually, Starch was grading the effectiveness of the ads (ie, whether or not they achieved their purpose of standing out in the subscriber's mind). This method of consumer reporting was called *aided recall*, popularly known as the *Starch test*. It was a successful strategy for moderately increasing the sale of newspapers and magazines. What Starch ultimately taught us was that to be a good market researcher one has to be a good psychologist.

The Starch test eventually became problematic with the changing of the times. First, Einstein's law of relativity (1907) disrupted classical Newtonian physics in which calculations were linearly based on the notion of a fixed point. Industry became affected as the new idea of multiple points of reference revolutionized technology. Starch's canvassing strategy, itself a linear construct, was too time consuming to keep up with the speed of the times.

Second, Starch's canvassing method relied on "warm-body" analysts for each consumer interviewed. The ratio of analysts to the growing subscriber base proved to be an unsustainable allocation of resources. There just were not enough hours in the day to gather and calculate data in a timely fashion.

Third, Ford's invention of the assembly line in 1914 increased the efficiency at which goods were produced (including the papers in the print industry). Again, Starch simply couldn't keep up the pace of the old canvassing method and stay relevant. He had to adjust, so he changed tactics by experimenting with radio advertising. The other lesson that Starch taught us is to be a relevant market researcher one has to keep up with the newer technologies.

UNAIDED RECALL

A younger contemporary of Starch was George Gallup (1901–1984), who became known as the *father of public polling* (The Gallup Poll). Gallup was not interested in print media, and he did not go door-to-door canvassing. That is probably because he was younger than Starch and exclusively developed his market research by polling consumers of the newer technologies of radio and television.

This was a difference in scope. Starch was interested in how to get more subscribers to buy newspapers and magazines. Gallup was interested in shaping public opinion, so he developed a poll algorithm for radio listeners and television viewers. His inventive method proved to be so successful that he was able to predict the 1936 presidential victory of Franklin D. Roosevelt over Alf Landon within a 4% margin of error. That was some accuracy for the times.

How was this accuracy possible? Gallup found a way to capture opinion polls that did not require warm-body mediators and visual prompting. Starch required customers to rely on memory. Gallup only required consumers to rely on sound (radio) and sight (television).

Gallup's form of polling eliminated the need for a canvasser to prompt customer memory and, instead, entirely trusted the consumer's emotional intelligence, although the consumer might not have been aware of it. Gallup's method was called *unaided recall* for this reason, and it trumped the Starch test.

THE ERA OF BIG BUSINESS: WHERE THE NETWORK IS KING

Radio and television advertising became a hit with consumers. The networks were able to extend the unaided advertising reach of businesses into any home that had a radio or television, and they required no more intervention than the subscriber's time for tuning in. The result was tremendous, and the networks benefited from the revenue streams that came in for exponentially increasing the bottom line of businesses that advertised on the networks. Consumer spending skyrocketed, and markets opened in places where none had existed. The next 70 years helped make the 20th century an era of consumerism.

Again, what facilitated the rise of consumerism was the networks. They were able to refine their ad copy simply by proliferating ads on the airwaves without having to physically canvas businesses to determine the effectiveness of their ads. The businesses reported on the effectiveness of the ads to the networks. Hence, the network databases grew as did their value in the eyes of competitive businesses who fought for advertising space.

It was not too long before the data analysts were able to interpret, track, predict, and even elicit buyer behavior for thousands of products and services nationwide with remarkable precision, but that precision came at a price. The networks, understanding the value they delivered to their highest-paying customers, restricted the supply of airtime only to those companies who could pay the ever-increasing rates. That meant more consumer data for the networks, and the highest-paying companies could effectively squash any competition and prohibit small businesses growth.

The Era of Small Business: Where the Relationship Is King

Because the larger businesses dominated the market, they were able to charge exorbitant prices for products and services that were not necessarily quality. In this, they lorded over the consumer who had little to no choice. Remember big business was working with large databases and did not have the emotional connection to their customers. Because small businesses far outnumbered the larger ones, it was a matter of survival for small business owners to figure out who their ideal customers were and how to reach them. Small business owners learned that they had the following natural advantages over their larger competitors:

- They better knew their customers' needs.
- Instead of making poor-quality products, they could create one high-quality product.
- They were better suited to serve the needs of locals.
- They could respond quickly to sudden economic changes.

The benefit of face-to-face interaction with real people was the creation of quality products and services scaled to the real-world and real-time needs of the consumer.

The larger companies did not seem to mind the attrition rate of customers at first because they were looking at the large numbers. However, with thousands of small businesses connecting with locals, it was too late when the large companies caught on to what was happening. Overleveraged and undermined, several notoriously successful companies and monopolies were forced to downsize, go bankrupt, or disappear altogether. Small business relationships became king.

THE INTERNET AND NICHE MARKETING: WHERE THE BRAND IS KING

Since the advent of the internet, the small business found itself having to get creative in order to stay relevant, stay visible, and keep its customers. Customer loyalty was no longer along traditional geographic lines, and the chasm between local and global brands shrank. Buyer behavior got so finicky that the invention of a new algorithm became necessary to reel in the apparent lawlessness that governed it. That new algorithm was marketing segmentation.

Marketing segmentation involves the following 4 factors:
1. Describing your customer according to his or her need
2. Identifying your customer's needs across a wide spectrum
3. Devising multiple advertising strategies that will effectively reach your customer
4. Delivering in the ways that your consumer needs you to deliver

In marketing segmentation, one designs a product or service that meets a consumer need across a wide spectrum of consumer types. Because these products and services are value propositions, the product or service becomes a rallying point—what is notably called a *brand*.

Brands are key to niche marketing because customers can contribute in the form of interactions such as customer comments, customer care lines, "likes," and "shares" on social media, among others.

In light of tradition, niche marketing is a backward way to build a brand. Traditionally, brands were built over decades by the unaided recall strategies mentioned earlier in this chapter, a term commonly called *push marketing* today. With push marketing, the business relentlessly saturates buyer space with its products and services.

Niche (brand) marketing uses pull marketing, which is a nonintrusive way of marketing in which brands are strategically "dripped" out to the consumer in order to appear casual. Such marketing acknowledges the exhaustion of the average consumer from being the target of multiple coercive marketing efforts. The hope of niche marketing is that the consumer finds the brand compelling and authentic.

TODAY THE CUSTOMER IS KING

Over the last few years, buyer behavior has slowly evolved once more. If one pays careful attention, it is obvious that the market has adjusted in favor of the consumer. It seems that the entire commercial world has been retrofitted for online convenience so that it is no longer necessary to leave one's house, stand in long lines, or interact with people. Most product purchases can be made on a smartphone and delivered in record time to any location of one's choice. This is beneficial to the consumer.

We have come full circle back to Starch and his warm-body contact with individual subscribers. Of course, it would be absurd to suggest canvassing neighborhoods for one's ideal consumer, but that begs the answer to the following question: "What was consumer behavior like before modern market research?"

That answer is so strikingly simple it is almost absurd.

- Consumers bought things that they needed from people they knew.
- Consumers bought enough of it to serve their purpose.
- Consumers maintained a relationship with the buyer in case they needed to get more.

What that translates into is simple: the consumer is king. Notice how consumer-centric each point is:

- The consumer has the need.
- The consumer fulfills his or her need.
- The consumer knows where to get his or her need fulfilled the next time.

THE HERO'S JOURNEY:
WHERE YOUR CUSTOMER IS THE HERO

In the classic adventure story, there are few main characters. There is usually one hero, a few of his sidekicks, a bad guy and his minions, and other background characters. In today's market, think about your customer as the hero of his or her own story.

Joseph Campbell wrote *The Hero With a Thousand Faces*[2] in which he analyzed the classic hero's journey story line, which virtually every culture has used to tell stories about its heroes overcoming an obstacle and winning notoriety.

I have reduced the template into 12 steps for simplification. Each step correlates to the numbers on a clock moving clockwise.

1:00: The hero is called to an adventure.

2:00: The hero meets a mentor.

3:00: The hero crosses the threshold into an unknown world.

4:00: The hero experiences a series of trials and failures.

5:00: The hero develops new skills through trial and error.

6:00: The hero dies and is reborn.

7:00: The hero has a startling revelation.

8:00: The hero finally "gets" the code to the unknown world.

9:00: The hero is changed.

10:00: The hero wins his or her "prize."

11:00: The hero returns home.

12:00: The hero enjoys the new normal.

In this market research fable, your customer is the hero of his or her own story. He or she is trying to do a good deed (despite opposition), make things right (as best he or she can), or return home (despite the obstacles). Your hero will buy from you if what you have to offer him or her helps to achieve his or her purpose, which is to become the hero.

When it comes to the eye care industry, your hero's need might look something like the following:

1:00: Your customer has an eye concern.

2:00: Your customer sees one of your advertisements or attends one of your seminars.

3:00: Your customer's eye concern gets worse, but he or she tries the lesser route.

4:00: Your customer experiences further complications.

5:00: Your customer begins to understand some of your advice (at 2:00).

6:00: The customer is at the end of his or her rope.

7:00: More of your information (2:00) makes sense to your customer.

8:00: Your customer finally makes the decision to use your product or services.

9:00: Your customer has great intentions to still use your product or services.

10:00: Your customer uses your product or service.

11:00: The customer returns home.

12:00: The customer enjoys his or her new vision.

This template seems easy enough, but it is actually more complicated than it looks. Your customers, as the heroes of their stories, are not thinking about you every day. They are not always remembering all of the important information from your seminar or their promise to follow up with you or the sense of concern they felt when they last spoke to you. Your customers have enough concerns, worries, and distractions in their own world that they are not going to pick up on all of the obvious cues for when they should be remembering your product or service.

Position Yourself by Becoming a Secondary Character

As an entrepreneur and business owner, you can find yourself so enthusiastic about your own products and services that you come across as a self-congratulatory and larger-than-life character—too large to play a secondary character in your customer's story. Remember there is only room for one hero and that is your customer.

Despite the best of intentions, if you believe that your product or service is exactly what your customers need, that is not enough to convince them. You need to honor their role as the hero by strategically positioning yourself as a complementary character. Making yourself a hero puts you in competition with your consumers, which can sabotage a product or service that your customers need.

Not all steps in the hero's journey are equal opportunities for targeting your customer. There are 3 opportunities in the 12 steps, and they correlate to the following 3 kinds of customers in our market research fable:

1. One needing a mentor (2:00)
2. One needing assistance (5:00)
3. One needing to be rescued (10:00)

Depending on where your potential customer is in his or her story will determine what position you are in to make him or her a customer:

- (2:00) Advisory: Perhaps your customer knows nothing about your product or service; yet, he or she attends a seminar of yours. You should position your messaging so that he or she buys now without all the information or he or she might recall your messaging later when it becomes imminently relevant to him or her. In this role, you are playing the mentor. You should trust that when the student is ready, the teacher will appear.

- (5:00) Companionship: Perhaps your customer experiences a failure relative to the product or service that you offered him or her at 2:00 but that he or she refused. If it should come to your attention, this is yet another point at which you (1) insist that he or she buys now or (2) offer him or her a one-on-one meeting in which you insist that he or she buys. In this role, you are playing the companion or helper, and you should be more insistent than at 2:00.

- (10:00) Rescuer: Perhaps your customer is in dire straits. In a moment of panic or vulnerability, he or she insists on your product or service. Because buying is predicated on emotional states, his or her emotional state will pass. As the rescuer, make it easy for your customer to buy from you.

In today's current market, the divergence between the brand as king (niche marketing) and the customer as king (consumer-facing marketing) is growing ever wider. What used to be called *relationship marketing* is passé to your customer in 2019 who does not have time to squeeze another relationship into his or her already hectic schedule. The general rule is as follows: Make it easy for your customer to get in and out. He or she will thank you for it.

By segmenting your customer base, branding your product or service as complementary to your customer's story, and positioning yourself to close your client when he or she is most emotionally ready, you will have the critical building blocks for building your customer base in this consumer-facing market.

REFERENCES

1.　Starch D. *Advertising: Its Principles, Practices, and Techniques.* Scott Foresman and Company; 1914.
2.　Campbell J. *The Hero With a Thousand Faces.* Pantheon Books; 1949.

The Patient Experience

Shareef Mahdavi, BA, CEEE

The great management scientist Peter Drucker famously said that "the aim of marketing is to make selling superfluous,"[1] implying that effective marketing would make the selling process unnecessary. Unfortunately, marketing by eye care practices has often been reduced to a single activity: advertising. Advertising itself is but one of many forms of paid promotion and can be effective, but rather than employing it strategically, many practices use advertising as the key driver for new patients. Although its value and effectiveness continue to be questioned by physicians and their accountants, advertising continues to be used. It remains thought of as the primary means of building the practice's brand to increase awareness and interest with a specific call to action that often includes some type of price incentive. One common example is "Call now to receive $500 off of LASIK!" Please ask yourself the following question: Would you be motivated to take action to save $500 on a life-changing procedure that involves surgery on your eyes when you know little about it or whether you are even a candidate?

Wang M, ed. *Grow Your Eye Care Practice: High-Impact Pearls From the Marketing Experts* (pp 35-44). © 2021 Taylor & Francis Group.

Indeed, price advertising has done more to harm rather than promote the laser vision correction category, but it is part of a larger problem when it comes to advertising of medical procedures, which is what happens next in the process. Think about what happens before you have guests come over to dinner in your home. You make sure the house is clean, and the meal is prepared in advance of the arrival of your guests. Everything should be in order. This principle is routinely violated when applied to typical advertising by ophthalmic practices because guests typically are invited to come over before the house is clean and ready. In this analogy, guests arrive and find the place to be a mess.

Sadly, this scenario happens frequently and can be illustrated by the way most practices answer the telephone. In studies conducted by SM2 Strategic to assess phone inquiries by prospective patients,[2] only 29% of practices achieved what was set as a reasonable standard that would motivate a patient to want to schedule a consultation. Recordings of the conversations (done with permission) revealed a lack of subject knowledge as well as reasonable telephone skills. Given that practices spend thousands of dollars each month in advertising designed to make the phone ring, these studies demonstrate that the house is still "messy," and the money is not well spent. Although leads are generated, they end up not being handled effectively, and the patient chooses either not to have the procedure or not to have it with that practice.

The problem does not go away for prospective patients who do visit the practice. They are often poorly greeted and asked to sit in a waiting room before being taken back. Tests are done, a consultation is performed, and a recommendation is made, only to have the patient conclude that he or she needs to think about it. Again, the money dedicated to promotional advertising was being spent before the practice had its customer service processes finely tuned to maximize the value (ie, result) of that spending.

INTERNAL VERSUS EXTERNAL MARKETING

As a marketing executive earlier in my career, I often advised practices to get their house in order before inviting people over. Focusing on operational processes to make sure that customer service basics are well handled is the top priority. After that, there is a wide range of activities that can be deployed to generate awareness and interest without committing to a large advertising budget, which collectively can be termed *internal marketing*. This distinction is helpful to define marketing activities that happen mainly inside the practice and target current patients as well as their network of family, friends, and colleagues.

In-office posters or brochures, webinars, patient testimonials, and direct mail or newsletters to current patients are all forms of internal marketing. This should again take priority over paid external marketing because it is far less costly. It is also far easier to reach this target audience given that a relationship has already been established. The ground here tends to be far more fertile ground than that beyond your doors.

Advertising, both literally and figuratively, is the last thing you should do. Marketing, although important, is only going to take the prospective patient to your front door. From there (and, as shown later, even before they arrive), the focus needs to be on making the patient's experience one that will help him or her move through the decision process and move forward with your recommendation.

CUSTOMER SERVICE VERSUS CUSTOMER EXPERIENCE

When it comes to elective medicine, the requirements for both customer service and customer experience are much higher than what has traditionally been offered in medical environments with third parties footing the bill. Patients are now paying customers; expectations are high both in terms of clinical outcome and the overall experience. In this context, patients are wearing their "customer" hat and tend to remember how they were treated far more vividly than what they paid or even their clinical outcome. This in part helps explain why doctors who are viewed as nice do not often get sued, even if their outcomes are not the best.

Many practices confuse customer service with customer experience. There is a difference. Service focuses on the operational components as activities that are performed and happen *to* the individual. Employees are typically evaluated on how well they perform their duties, which include an element of customer service. When employees take extra care, a patient may say they provided great service. When failures occur, which are inevitable in a service-related business, we say the customer suffered from poor service.

On the other hand, experience is a larger dynamic that includes customer service. Experiences are inherently personal; they take place inside the individual. The level of service provided is just one component of the overall experience. Customer service has evolved from being viewed as the complaint-handling department (people of a certain age will recall the window in the back of the department store) to a more fully integrated function in companies across virtually every industry that sells to consumers. Although having strong customer service is now a standard for most businesses, health care and medical practices are just now catching up in this regard, with patient experience being synonymous with customer experience.

Most practices (and indeed most businesses) tend to overestimate how well we are doing in customer service as perceived and defined by the customer. This happens because (1) only a small percentage of patients with issues actually say something and (2) we have an overinflated sense of how good we perform in this regard. A good example of this second point came out of a survey of 300 leading chief executive officers,[3] 80% of whom rated their customer service as excellent. A follow-up survey involving the customers of the companies led by these chief executive officers tells a different story because only 8% of customers collectively rated the customer service as excellent.

Many medical practices have begun to focus on customer service, understanding that their patients are also their customers. Furthermore, they understand that protocols to define what should happen when the patient is "vertical" are just as critical as those that are deployed during testing or surgery when the patient is "horizontal." Even with this focus, doctors and administrators can become complacent when they see weekly reports showing patients are generally satisfied or have not recently seen a major complaint:

Q: What is the easiest way to create a memorable experience?

A: Poor service!

This riddle helps illustrate why, in the pre-internet era, if you have great service at a restaurant you will tell 3 people; yet, if the service is poor, you will tell 10. With the advent of review sites such as Yelp, a complaint about poor service is amplified to reach a much larger audience. This reality of how rapidly bad news spreads creates an imperative for practices to focus on getting their service basics under control. The dining out equivalent to this looks like the following:

- Customers are seated promptly.
- Customers are greeted by waiter or waitress.
- Food arrives on time, is hot, and tastes good.

There was a point in time when these services would warrant a rave review because the standards for dining were not what they are today. Today, systems are in place, and staff are trained to make sure all of these things happen and the service is good. However, good service does not have the same value as a memorable experience.

BRANDING AND EXPERIENCE

If you pay attention to advertising these days, you will see a lot of companies tout the experience they offer, attempting to use whatever focus they have on customer experience as a differentiating factor. In my opinion, this is a mistake, and it is far better to allow people to conclude that they had a great experience on the back end rather than try to set the expectation for this on the front end. *The Experience Economy*[4] coauthor Joseph Pine reinforces this point when he explains that "a brand is simply the promise of a future experience" (personal communication, oral, October 1996). Companies that enjoy strong brand reputation among customers often have earned this because of the experience people have when engaging with the company and not because it was signaled as part of a promotional message. Whether shopping for computers (Apple), driving a new car (Tesla), or staying at a hotel (Four Seasons), people pay more for brands they like, and people pay even more when the experience they have reinforces their desire for the brand. One thing for sure is that these experiences are not accidental but rather extremely well planned and executed.

The principles of customer experience used by leading brands are available to the medical practice. In the next section, the concept of customer experience and how it can be put into practice in your practice are explored.

THE ROLE OF EXPERIENCE

To take Peter Drucker's quote a step further, the goal of customer experience should be to make marketing superfluous. As stated by authors Pine and Gilmore[5] in their original *Harvard Business Review* article, "the experience *is* the marketing." The authors believe that greater economic value can be derived through the intentional staging of experiences and that a long-term shift in our economy is taking place.[5] A year later, they published *The Experience Economy*,[4] which is now in its second edition. It is a breakthrough in understanding both what is happening in the world and how businesses and organizations can maintain their competitive edge by focusing on customer experience. As services are becoming automated, commoditized, and thus seen as less valuable, we see the rise of experiences as a distinct form of economic output, leading to greater economic growth in the same manner that services eventually supplanted manufacturing of goods as the dominant form of economic activity in developed nations. This repeated an earlier process in which manufacturing

Figure 5-1. The value of a cup of coffee increases exponentially in the shifts from commodity to goods, goods to services, and services to experiences.

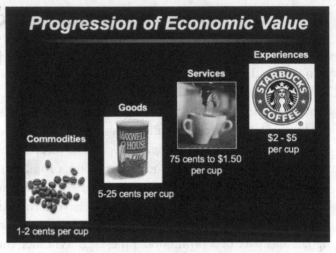

Figure 5-2. The value of vision correction increases as it moves through the economic progression. Because LASIK is inherently transformational, many practices ignored the experiential aspect of the offering, which led to commoditization.

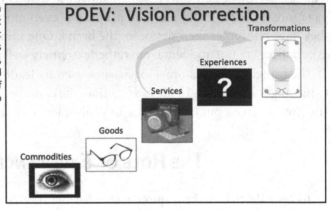

overtook farming as agriculture underwent increasing efficiency and automation, temporarily displacing workers.

Their foundational model, called the progression of economic value[5] (POEV), is illustrated in Figure 5-1. This demonstrates what has happened to coffee in terms of the increase in value over time. A cup of coffee, valued in pennies as a commodity, extracts far greater value when it is part of Starbucks or other premium, experience-driven coffee retailers.

The POEV model can be applied to numerous industry categories, and vision correction surgery provides another compelling example as shown in Figure 5-2. In working to help increase the value of laser vision correction, both economically and as perceived by customers, I postulate that the experiential aspects surrounding the procedure have been largely ignored because surgeons were comfortable performing a service (LASIK surgery) that was

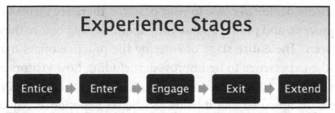

Figure 5-3. The 5E model, developed in 1997 by the architectural firm Doblin, divided customer experience into 5 distinct stages, each of which presents an opportunity for medical practices.

inherently transformational for the customer. A transformational experience, such as LASIK, is one that is so unique that it changes the customer from before to after. The POEV model can also help explain what happened with the attempt to commoditize LASIK. The transformational nature of the procedure was so powerful that it caused LASIK surgeons and staff to ignore the experiential components of the offering, leaning too heavily on the technology and the outcome.

In customer experience, 2 key measurements of success are the amount of time and money the consumer is spending with you. The opportunity for consumers to spend thousands of dollars of their money on an elective procedure is one that should never be taken for granted, and the perception of value that can be created through a well-designed experience can serve to boost reputation, referral patterns, and revenue.

STAGES OF EXPERIENCE

Chicago architectural design firm Doblin developed the 5E model for compelling experiences[6] showing the customer experience across 5 distinct stages, each one offering an opportunity for the experience-minded practice to design aspects that help form a unique and memorable experience overall for the patient (Figure 5-3).

Most people think of customer experience only in terms of when customers are physically present, such as during the LASIK consultation or the day of surgery. Although that encounter serves as the main event, the experience begins long before, starting with their visit to your website as well as any contact with you or your staff before they ever come to the practice. This is part of the *entice* stage and, as noted earlier, is ripe for improvement both in the level of service as well as how the experience can be designed. Websites are often the entry point in the experience, and the digital experience is just as essential as what happens in person.

When patients decide to come to your practice, there are forms to complete, a check-in process, and perhaps some time spent waiting before they are taken back to be seen. The entire stage of *entering* the practice offers many opportunities for the experience to be improved, including how visitors are greeted and welcomed, what is available for them to do while they wait, and how the office space is designed so that it lends to a better experience. My own bias is that practices would be well served to eliminate the waiting room altogether, replacing it with a space that better uses customers' time and can also serve to reinforce the experience that the practice wants patients to have.

The fourth stage, known as *exit*, is similarly ripe for improvement. Perhaps there is a goodbye ritual that can be designed in which patients feel truly appreciated for trusting their vision with your practice. As with the entering stage, this is an often-neglected part of the experience.

Finally, the last stage is *extend* and is meant to prolong all the good feelings that took place when the patient was present, such as what takes place in the day 1 postoperative visit after LASIK. This last stage of experience can be viewed as activities designed to increase the memorability of the experience. Sometimes it comes in the form of memorabilia, which at the most basic level could be a T-shirt or mug emblazoned with the practice name. A bit higher up the experience chain would be a picture of the patient while at the practice, sent as part of a thank you card. Any type of gathering for alumni would be considered a way to extend the experience.

Taken as a sequence, a practice that is serious about making customer experience part of their strategy should look at every aspect that can be reimagined and improved. This means every patient encounter, every form, every physical space, and every piece of communication. To date, I have not visited a practice that did not yield opportunity to improve.

What About the Employee Experience?

We have often heard the refrains "the customer is always right" and "the customer is king." Although these sayings were intended to help businesses increase their focus on meeting customer needs, they do not always hold true. Leading restaurateur Danny Meyer, most recently known for his Shake Shack concept, rates customers as the second most important stakeholder after employees.[7] In essence, he is recognizing that it takes employees to make sure customers have a great experience. If the employees are not led and managed as the most valuable asset to the enterprise, customers will suffer. This single point is what I predict will prevent most medical practices from successfully integrating customer experience so that it becomes an effective differentiator.

However, in practices that embrace their employees and strive to create a culture that empowers, respects, and rewards the desired employee behavior, a foundation exists that can have a major positive effect on how patients perceive their experience as customers of the practice. One of the best examples I have observed is at Vance Thompson Vision, which started in Sioux Falls, South Dakota, and has now expanded with locations in 5 states. As a practice that started with 2 employees in 1991, there are now just shy of 200 employees in what Dr. Thompson describes as his "work family," where communication is key to enabling the team to stage and deliver a meaningful experience for each and every patient. With a mission to be "the best on Earth," employee meetings take place on a daily basis (called the *holy huddle*) as well as via regular retreats.

Practice chief executive officer Matt Jensen[8] leads the employee team and is quick to describe how hard it is to make the experience appear seamless, with a great deal of training, coaching, and ongoing development handled by his team of leaders who handle one or more areas of the practice. The customer experience requires a daily focus and a long-term commitment. It is not a quick fix that can be used to boost short-term results but instead an investment in people. A lot is expected of the employees who work at Vance Thompson Vision, and their reward extends beyond their paycheck to a larger sense of purpose in helping people improve their eyesight and the way they see the world. Their practice serves as an example of what is possible in ophthalmology when the practice treats the patients as if they are also customers and also treats the staff as the most valuable resource in delivering the desired experience.

CONCLUSION

As a strategy to differentiate the ophthalmic practice, customer experience has the ability to exceed what can be achieved vs a marketing strategy that focuses on differentiating via the technology used, the skill of the surgeon, or price in terms of fees charged for elective procedures. Each one of these can be replicated over time by other practices. Customer experience is unique in that it becomes part of the fabric and cultural DNA of the practice. Even if other competing practices came to observe what was taking place, it is highly unlikely that they will be able to copy and replicate what was achieved. There is simply too much work and effort that goes into planning and implementing the desired experience that it does not translate well to a different practice with a different set of norms and values. Indeed, competing practices would do well to define their own customer experience for their patients and strive to have an offering that is unique and memorable to patients all on its own.

As with marketing, patient experience is an area in which the practice should strive to continuously improve and avoid concluding that the job is done. Experiences need to be refreshed and upgraded as consumer sensibility evolves over time.

REFERENCES

1. Drucker PF. *The Essential Drucker*. Harper Collins Publishers; 2001:21.
2. Mahdavi S. Telephone improvement project: a skills assessment of refractive surgery providers. Pleasanton, CA: SM2 Consulting; 2006.
3. DiJulius J. *What's the Secret? To Providing a World-Class Customer Experience*. Wiley Publishing; 2008:17-19.
4. Pine J, Gilmore J. *The Experience Economy*. Harvard Business School Press; 1999.
5. Pine J, Gilmore J. Welcome to the experience economy. *Harvard Business Review*. July-August 1998:97-105.
6. About Doblin. Doblin: A Deloitte Business. Updated 2020. Accessed August 3, 2020. https://doblin.com/about
7. Cutrone C. Danny Meyer to 'Treps: put your employees first, customers will follow. The founder debunked the myth of "the customer is always right" at Inc.'s latest Business Owners Council event last night in New York City. *Inc.* Published January 28, 2014. Accessed September 8, 2020. https://www.inc.com/carolyn-cutrone/danny-meyer-speaks-at-inc-business-owners-council.html
8. Mahdavi S. "This is the Super Bowl of leadership" [video]. YouTube. Published April 24, 2020. Accessed September 8, 2020. https://www.youtube.com/watch?v=sTkSMITiDCA&t=382s

6

Branding Versus Call to Action

Tracy Schroeder Swartz, OD, MS, FAAO, Dipl ABO and Ming Wang, MD, PhD

When planning your marketing strategy, there is a difference between a branding campaign and a call-to-action campaign. The goal of a branding campaign is to develop an image, increase awareness, and promote positive thoughts for your practice. It has more history with traditional advertising media such as radio and television and is used less with digital media.[1] An immediate response is not the main goal but may prompt the audience to go to a website or contact the office for more information. Advertisements that do not contain contact information are typically well established, extremely well known, and greatly appreciated by the audience. The goal is to promote the practice as a whole and to keep your practice in the forefront, so when people need eye care or decide to pursue a certain treatment, they contact your office over the competition. If you build a strong reputation as a practice, they may not run out the door this minute, but they will when they need your services.

A call-to-action campaign is designed to encourage the target audience to do something immediately. Examples include short-term price reductions, or

Wang M, ed. *Grow Your Eye Care Practice:*
High-Impact Pearls From the Marketing Experts (pp 45-50).

sales in the retail world, and new product launches announcing a new technology or new doctor to the practice. The goal is to entice the audience to contact the office or do something immediately. In the retail world, an example is an offer for 0% financing on a new vehicle purchased by the end of the month from dealer inventory. In the eye care world, an example would be to respond to a radio commercial or email sent to targeted patients for a promotional intense pulsed light treatment package before Friday. In addition to determining the type of campaign, you must also determine the best media outlet to use for your campaign.

Costs

The media chosen will often determine the costs, with television being the most expensive and social media being the least. Tracking that investment cost is easier with social media than with traditional advertising. With television and radio, the patient would need to report seeing the advertisement or hearing it on the radio. For example, the advertisement might tell the patient to say a certain phrase to tag the source. A newspaper advertisement could include instructions to bring the ad to the office or clip a coupon.

Tracking with online advertising is much easier because the ads can track "click-through" rates. When the audience sees a digital ad, they are instructed to "click here" to be taken to the office website. This can be easily tracked. Instagram, Twitter, and Facebook can direct the audience to the website's landing page, or a specific page, such as dry eye treatments, vision correction surgery, or contact lenses.

Advertising to build the brand is more difficult to track because the patient is less likely to report one ad in particular upon presenting to the office. The office tagline might become so familiar that people refer to it in the office or, even better, in public. However, it is difficult to know what media expense is best for this plan.

To Coupon or Not to Coupon

Some feel reducing the price for services reduces the value of the service or reduces the importance of the brand. In these cases, using incentives to entice patients may not be the preferred option. If paying a higher price means getting a higher product, brand advertising may be a better choice.

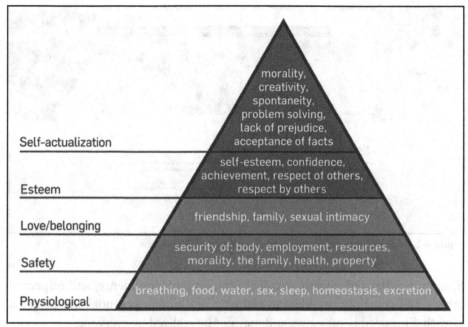

Figure 6-1. Maslow's hierarchy of needs. Needs required for survival are lower in the pyramid, whereas more emotional needs are located higher. (Reprinted with permission via Creative Commons Attribution-ShareALike 3.0 Unported. Factoryjoe.)

Step 1: Branding

Most marketeers would suggest building the brand. The audience needs to recognize the name, the logo, and the chosen "face" of the practice. This may be the lead doctor, the location, the building, the services offered, or the specialty if the only one in town. Here, the story is told, and the seed is planted so to speak.

Discuss why patients should visit you. Educate the audience on why you are preferred over the competition. Be seen in the community promoting your services.

Note that consumers build the brand not the company. Consumers develop perceptions of the company and have expectations for the brand.[2] Companies reinforce these opinions by delivering what the consumer expects. The foundation of brand building is considering what consumers (ie, your patients) need. When they feel that need should be fulfilled, your brand should come to their mind.

In 1943, Abraham Maslow wrote *A Theory of Human Motivation*. He identified 5 human needs ranked in a hierarchy (Figure 6-1).[2] Physiological needs include those things people need to survive. Safety needs include things that give us a sense of security such as personal health, family, and a job. Love and belonging needs are those humans have related to family, relationships, and friendships.

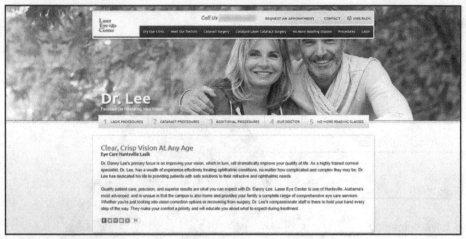

Figure 6-2. A website focusing on building the reputation of the practice.

Esteem includes self-esteem, personal achievement, confidence, and respect of others. Self-actualization refers to realizing full human potential and personal growth. This need is subjective and may not be realized by everyone.

As you move upward in this hierarchy, needs become less essential for survival and more emotional. If you consider each level of need for your target audience and develop marketing communications to address those needs for consumers, you should be more successful. Marketing communications must differentiate your product from your competition and position it as the only solution (Figure 6-2).

Step 2: Call to Action

Once the brand is established, harvesting of the crops you previously planted occurs. Be proactive in planning, and consider what services tend to be more popular at certain times of the year. For example, vision correction procedures tend to peak in January and December, whereas pediatric services peak before school starts. Jewelry stores advertise their brand all year but will use call-to-action advertisements around Valentine's Day, Mother's Day, and Christmas.

Psychology to consider when planning a call-to-action campaign is Aristotle's 7 causes of human action[2]:

1. Chance: Do not leave your target audience unguided or leave their contacting you to chance. Educate them regarding your brand.
2. Nature: Both human nature and environmental nature are important to motivate consumers to act. Ensure the actions you tell your target audience to take align with their natures.

3. Compulsion: In a world of instant gratification, compulsion causes a significant amount of people to do things because things are quick and easy. Facilitating your target audience to act will increase conversion rates.

4. Habit: Many daily habits are subconscious but play a role in when people act. Setting expectations and consistently meeting consumer expectations develops trust in your brand and leads to action.

5. Reason: The reason may be rational or irrational. Rational thinking applies more to lower levels of the hierarchy of needs, whereas irrational applies to the higher levels of needs. Higher-level needs require marketers to develop perceived reasons for consumers to take action in their favor by appealing to emotions.

6. Passion: Passion is also related to emotions. If you identify the emotion to encourage someone to take action, he or she will be more likely to complete the action.

7. Desire: If you understand what the target audience wants or needs, you can encourage the audience to desire what you offer. It is more about a lifestyle or personal benefit, goal, or want than a need.

If these traits are addressed in your call to action, the campaign will likely be more successful.

Once you determine how to target the audience with a message, the media is chosen. The following are suggestions to include in your call to action[3]:

- Make them action oriented.
- Use persuasive text.
- Include strong visuals.
- Create a sense of urgency.
- Make them easy to find.

Action words should be used to command the audience to act (Figure 6-3). The offer should be clear and detailed to reduce confusion. Enable a direct connection via the website link, phone number, or mobile application. Ask the audience to perform one task only to accomplish your goal. Rather than using "Call us to sign up for a free consultation" and "Visit our website and sign up for a free consultation," use "Sign up for a free consultation by phone or on our website."[4] Time limits or limiting the number of offerings encourages the audience to act quickly. Address fears by addressing them directly, such as "Call now to learn more about modern vision correction procedures." Bright colors and dynamic graphics will capture the audience's attention. Do not overcrowd the page so the offer is difficult to find. Use a 20% larger font than the background text information to make the offer stand out.

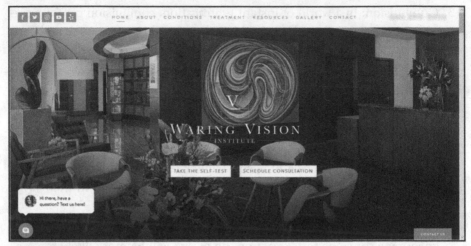

Figure 6-3. An example of call to action on a site landing page. The chat option, self-test enticement, scheduling option, and contact option are easily visible and all located above the scroll level on the page. (Reprinted with permission from the Waring Vision Institute.)

Another thing to consider with call-to-action campaigns is you are asking the audience to do something. If you ask someone to do something every time you see him or her, that person will likely tune you out or take the stairs if he or she sees you in the elevator. Telling the story of the brand must be combined with periodic call-to-action ads. Again, some feel call-to-action advertising reduces the quality of the brand and rarely use it at all. Premier practices may reserve call-to-action campaigns for educational events such as seminars or product launches.

References

1. Proud Media. What is the difference between a branding and call to action? Published February 10, 2014. Accessed August 4, 2020. http://www.proudmedia.com.au/difference-branding-call-action/

2. Gunelius S. The psychology and philosophy of branding, marketing, needs, and actions. Published March 5, 2014. Accessed August 4, 2020. https://www.forbes.com/sites/work-in-progress/2014/03/05/the-psychology-and-philosophy-of-branding-marketing-needs-and-actions/#1514e8d9725a

3. Sukhraj R. Call-to-action examples: 17 designed to earn clicks and generate leads [Updated for 2020]. Published November 29, 2019. Accessed August 4, 2020. https://www.impactbnd.com/blog/examples-of-calls-to-action-for-lead-generation

4. Printwand. 14 tips for writing the best call to action (with examples). Published January 2, 2013. Accessed August 4, 2020. https://www.printwand.com/blog/14-tips-for-writing-the-best-call-to-action-with-examples

7

Word of Mouth
How Can We Encourage Our Patients to Refer?

Catherine Maley, MBA

A word-of-mouth referral is the absolute best advertisement you can incorporate into your practice. It is also the cheapest form of advertising that you can invest in, and it takes minimal time and effort.

We all know the best patient is a referred patient. When a friend tells another friend, family member, or colleague about you, that is golden. They are already presold on you, they are not as price sensitive, and they are more likely to stay loyal to you. Word-of-mouth referrals will increase your closing ratios, decrease your external marketing costs, and grow your practice. So, how do you get them?

Word of mouth referrals do not just happen. They must be deserved, encouraged, and sought after using creative, subtle methods. Sure, you will get some referrals from your core group of fans in your practice (every practice has them), but you want them from every patient, not just the chosen few.

Wang M, ed. *Grow Your Eye Care Practice:*
High-Impact Pearls From the Marketing Experts (pp 51-56).
© 2021 Taylor & Francis Group.

You grow your word-of-mouth referrals by focusing on them. Make word-of-mouth referrals a priority in your office; set up processes and incorporate strategies to obtain them.

REFERRALS START WITH FIVE-STAR CUSTOMER SERVICE

The easiest way to get patients talking about you is to give them something great to talk about. Offer extraordinary customer service to stand out. Of course, you need commitment from your staff to make patient satisfaction your number one priority. Nothing is more important than patient relations if you want to build a referral practice, so meet with your staff regularly to ensure they understand the importance of treating each patient with a warm and friendly attitude each time he or she calls or visits. Also, be sure your telephone is answered by the third ring, call back when you say you will, and do not keep patients waiting. Respect your patients' time and concerns, and they will brag about you to their friends.

COMPUTER TRACKING

You cannot really know who your advocates are unless you can track them accurately. It is vital that you have a computer system that automatically tracks referral sources so you know who is really referring people and who just says they will but never gets around to it. You also want to track who actually books procedures from these referrals. Good computer systems will outline in detail who referred who and the outcome in terms of revenues generated.

TALK TO YOUR PATIENTS

Referrals come from connecting with your patients so they feel cared about as people first and then as patients. Before you jump right into the medical reason they are there to see you about, spend a couple of minutes on them as people. Ask them about their family, their occupation, or anything else that strikes you as interesting from their patient intake forms.

When talking to patients, use their name and make eye contact with them. Ask them questions and then let them talk. The point is to bond with them personally first so they know you care about them. They will relax, open up to you, and talk more about themselves. You can learn so much about patients if you show you are interested in them. When doing so, you will be surprised what you learn. Perhaps they are members of the media or they are part of large companies that could use your services as an employee perk.

Consider this. Each of us has on average an inner circle of approximately 250 people. This inner circle includes friends, family, colleagues, neighbors, etc. If each of your patients only told 5 of his or her inner circle about you and those 5 people told 5 additional people, how quickly could you grow your practice?

Remember that like-minded people hang around with other like-minded people. You want your preferred patients to bring their friends to you. Do not take that for granted. Be sure to tell your patients that you want more patients just like them. Tell them if they send their friends, family, and colleagues to you, you promise to take good care of them.

NETWORK

I have watched physicians grow their practices quickly with networking. Remember the following adage: "It's not what you know, it's who you know." If you are good at networking, you can tap into groups of people who can become your preferred patients. Every person you meet should know who you are, what you do, and the services you offer. If nothing else, be sure your card says it so you can at least introduce yourself and hand him or her a card.

Look at who you know in your community. Perhaps you are friendly with the dentist down the hall or other noncompeting specialties who would be happy to refer their patients to you and vice versa. This can be done informally by exchanging business cards and handing them to the patients who need your services.

Perhaps your staff regularly visits a certain hair salon or works out at the popular gym nearby, or your office manager goes to yoga classes down the block. You can turn those casual alliances into viable word-of-mouth referral outlets by having your staff talk and then introduce you to the owners. If you hit it off, you can give them cards or a customized poster to display in their location, and, in return, you can give them a special price to offer their clients, customers, or patients.

GET INVOLVED IN YOUR COMMUNITY

Giving back to your community shows you care about the people living within it. Getting involved in a worthy cause makes you feel good, and it is good for the community. If you do not have a cause close to your heart and need to find something, think strategically.

If you want to be known as the *eye doc* in your community, perhaps you can offer your services to sports teams. If you want to get into the "in" social crowd in your community, work with the socialites in your area who give considerable time and money to a specific cause and get to know them. Become part of their crowd, and they will loyally go to you and send their like-minded friends to you as well.

USE CONTENT TO SPREAD THE WORD

Content is king on the internet so produce lots of it for different media channels so your patients can share it with their friends and new prospective patients can find you on their own. For example, you can videotape a consultation with a prospective patient talking about LASIK (with the patient's permission of course) and then upload it to YouTube and Vimeo. Break it down into small pieces and upload to Instagram video. Use the video screenshot in your Facebook banner ads that click to the full video with "Click Here to Schedule a Complimentary Consultation."

That is not all you can do with the video. Transcribe the patient consultation and use it for your blog posts, articles, and press releases. Send an email announcing it to your current patient list and add "Share this with a friend." The point is to cross-purpose one piece of content to many different media channels to increase your presence online.

SOCIAL MEDIA BOOTH

Make it fun and easy for your patients to share you with their friends on social media. Order a customized pop-up backdrop with your logo printed on it. Have it standing in a corner of your office near checkout. The patient can take pictures with you and your staff. They can videotape a testimonial and then upload it to their Facebook, Instagram, and Snapchat pages. Remember to obtain photo/video permission if you use this media for your marketing campaign.

EDUCATIONAL EVENTS WORTH TALKING ABOUT

Prospective patients may have researched eye procedures online, but they have not heard you personally describe procedures so grab your iPad (Apple) and shoot a couple informal videos explaining in your own words the benefits of the procedure as well as the process.

You can also do an online presentation using Zoom or GoToWebinar (LogMeIn, Inc) and PowerPoint (Microsoft) slides explaining procedures and include a call to action at the end, such as a complimentary consultation to encourage them to take the next step.

Invite your current patients to attend the seminar and have them invite their friends. Record the seminar to create content for your website and other internet marketing so prospective patients find you more easily.

THANK YOUR PATIENTS

Do not take referrals for granted. You want to thank your patients; however, a boring computer-generated form does not cut it. Patients want to be appreciated for their trust and acknowledged for their support so show them thanks. The following are examples of how to show your gratitude:

- Have your staff call them immediately to thank them.
- Write a personal note from you to thank them.
- Call them yourself to thank them.
- Send a gift of appreciation.

Behavior that is rewarded is repeated, so make a statement out of how much you appreciate their referral to encourage more referrals.

FREQUENT REFERRAL PROGRAM

Reward, encourage, and acknowledge those special patients who offer multiple referrals. Every practice has those patients who just love them! They visit often, and they know the names of the staff members' children and what schools they go to. They may live in the same neighborhood or attend the same school as your children. They go to your health club or play club sports with your family. You have a special group of loyal patients who sing your praises all over town. Whenever the subject of eye care comes up, they are the first to jump in and tell everyone what you have done for them and how happy they are with your care. These people can give out your number if they have a pen. If they do not, they will email your name, phone number, and address the next day.

Like everything else in life, 80% of the referrals will come from 20% of your patients. You can help those stats by going a step further. You can implement a frequent referral program, but do it with caution. You do not want to get into the game of giving away services if they refer so many people to you. Those patients who are trying to get deals from you by sending in their friends may be more trouble than they are worth. They may send you patients you do not want and may be in it for the wrong reasons. You want the patients who are truly ecstatic about you and want to sing your praises, not those who just want a break on their eye procedure.

ASK

Any written communications coming from you should remind the audience how much you appreciate referrals. Add the phrase "Bring a Friend" to your invitations and "Send This to a Friend" on your website and internet messages. Add a special note in your blog posts and advertising. Display an eye-catching reminder sign in your reception area. Include referral cards in your correspondence to your patients to encourage them to spread their appreciation. The more your patients are reminded, the more they will remember you when they are speaking with their friends.

THE GOLDEN RULE

Patients have to be truly happy and satisfied with their result as well as the service they received to brag about you to their friends and family. Be sure every single patient has a "WOW" experience every time they are in contact with you, your staff, and your office and watch your referrals grow.

Alignment of a Marketing and Sales Strategy

Kane Harrison

There is little doubt that a cohesive marketing strategy equals more sales, but it is certainly easier said than done. There is so much that falls on the shoulders of marketers and sellers in eye care services today. The world is moving as fast as our culture can push it, and we now have an ever-shifting consumer focus.

Physician business leaders are required to focus on many moving parts in the day-to-day operations of an eye care practice. These may include juggling C-suite–level decisions around operations, marketing, finance, and human resources while conducting consultations and performing highly sophisticated surgeries with the now educated public expecting often better than perfect outcomes. One element you can change in your business that will have measurable results is to build a strong culture and drive revenue. This chapter shows how you can align your marketing and sales strategy and push your business to a new level.

Aligning your marketing and sales strategy seems incredibly obvious. However, it is rarely implemented because it is often more complicated

Wang M, ed. *Grow Your Eye Care Practice: High-Impact Pearls From the Marketing Experts* (pp 57-64).

than appreciated. Most fail because they focus only on the mechanical aspects of sales and marketing (advertorial positioning, content, and messaging) and neglect the cultural (objective communication, data-driven analysis, and cohesive directional and critical thinking) change that must take place between the marketing and sales teams to perform at high levels. All of this is paramount when you become focused on a results-driven marketing and sales strategy. The focus on the mechanical aspect of marketing will produce the typical blurred results of traditional marketing that has been ingrained in those marketing ophthalmology. Once the cultural aspect is introduced and married to your thinking, you can focus your marketing on a result like a defined return on investment, an attended consultation, or completed surgery. To do this, you need to teach your marketing and sales leaders to think like business owners rather than employees. When you are a business owner, revenue matters. Employees tend to lose sight of how money turns up in their bank account each week. This is not the fault of the employee. It is the residual effect of antiquated thinking passed down from an antiquated system. This is a strategy I have been using for many years, and it is the only way forward for those marketing eye care. In fact, it is the future of marketing and sales in general. It is often said that the best way to look forward is to evaluate the past.

One of the founding principles of modern marketing and advertising is known as AIDA. The acronym stands for Attention, Interest, Desire (or Decision), and Action. It is often said that if your marketing or advertising is missing just 1 of the 4 AIDA steps, it will fail.

American advertising and sales pioneer Elias St. Elmo Lewis, a legend in the industry, coined the phrase and the approach. As far back as 1899, Lewis preached "attract attention, awaken interest, persuade and convince." In his article "Catch-Line and Argument," Lewis postulated at least 3 principles to which an advertisement should conform:

> The mission of an advertisement is to attract a reader, so that he will look at the advertisement and start to read it; then to interest him, so that he will continue to read it; then to convince him, so that when he has read it he will believe it. If an advertisement contains these three qualities of success, it is a successful advertisement.[1(p124)]

It is not far from the AIDA model now used around the world. Although Lewis was certainly thinking ahead of his time, I am not certain he could have predicted the pace at which our culture is evolving nor could he have foreseen the advancements in technology and communication. Although the model itself is much the same, how consumers move through it has changed dramatically.

Begin the alignment of the marketing strategy with your sales strategy by defining the terms *marketing* and *sales*. Marketing is the activity, set of institutions, and processes for creating, communicating, delivering, and exchanging offerings that have value for customers, clients, partners, and society at large. Sales is the exchange of a commodity for money; it is the action of selling something.

Sales teams often complain about how hard it is to sell what marketers present to be sold, and marketers complain about the lack of performance from the sales team. This is a familiar situation in many businesses. In the past, marketing teams would use content to get people interested in products and services through a number of traditional outlets, such as billboards, television, radio, and newspapers. They would usually have a strong call to action accompanied with branding, and sales would take over early in the process. Both teams would continue on their separate ways.

The consumer focus shift has aided digital content marketing's rise to prominence and overall effectiveness. There is now at least one piece of content for every stage in the sales funnel. Relevant content has become the best sales tool for the sales team. For this shift to translate into a measurable result, several important things need to happen.

Sales and marketing teams require an efficient means of communication. There should be a clear method of requesting projects and getting access to internal information. Cloud-based programs like Slack (Slack Technologies, Inc; www.slack.com) and Basecamp (www.basecamp.com) have become part of the second tier of communication in high-functioning businesses. Relying on email communication for tracking progress between teams will tip the scales toward failure. If you are not in a position to move to a Salesforce–type cloud-based solution (Salesforce.com, Inc; www.salesforce.com) that will integrate your programs through an application programming interface (ie, application programming interfaces just allow applications to communicate with one another), programs like Slack that can be accessed and monitored from anywhere will prove to be a saving grace for your teams and anyone overseeing the strategy.

The marketing team needs to have a clear understanding of how the sales process works, including how salespeople talk to clients and what resources they are currently using. The misstep marketers often make is not taking advantage of how much the sellers know about the product. It is one thing to market to a persona. It is another to talk to your salespeople who intimately know and understand your patients and their challenges.

The sales team must have a clear understanding of the strengths and creativity of the marketing team. They should be able to help prioritize projects and provide feedback on the content's performance. A misstep sellers often make is not trusting marketing to drive those important brand awareness conversations. A strong marketing department can help sellers be more efficient and focus much more on high-value activities, but that can mean letting go of the traditional top of the sales funnel activities such as early phone calls, emails, and text messaging and allowing marketing to put good leads in their lap.

All team members should understand the individual goals in the sales funnel and the expected result of the overall strategy. Encourage both teams to discuss the strategy at the macrolevel early in the process to help each division negate any foreseeable pitfalls. The following should be discussed:

- Build a strategy reflecting the stages of the patient's buying journey through the sales pipeline. Investigate this journey to bond the sales and marketing teams' thinking. Get the teams working together early in this process.

- Consider the rates of conversion. Pinpoint the conversion stages to determine potential patient tripping points. Tripping points in a sales funnel can be a sales team's nightmare.

- Take into consideration the time lag in decision making. Do not give the potential patient a reason to stop moving through the funnel; be clear in your communication and with any indirect information, such as handouts, so that your sales funnel continues to motivate the decision-making process.

- Ultimately, the decision to move forward with a procedure should always be that of the patients. It is the responsibility of your sales team to remove as many subjective decision motivators as they can so that patients, along with their physicians, can make an objective medical decision.

- Ninety percent of purchases are elective decisions. Potential patients need to be reminded why they need to purchase at every touch. People rarely ask questions during a captivating story, so take potential patients on a journey.

- Reflect on the contributions of both sales and marketing to generating revenues and gaining new patients.

The next stage is to create a focused pipeline model and use it to determine the objectives for each step of the individual campaigns. Each campaign should have specific goals for both sales and marketing. This is often where the divide is most felt between the marketing and sales teams. It is paramount for each team to use objective communication and object, supportive data at this point to maintain alignment. This is not the time for subjective communication or creative input that can become divisive. The individual campaigns should be integrated into a timeline, including suggested time frames and the responsibilities of the marketing and sales teams.

CHECKLIST FOR PRIORITIZING AREAS OF IMPROVEMENT

The following is a checklist that can be reviewed in order to prioritize areas needing improvement. The checklist will serve as the groundwork for an effective marketing strategy that will stay in alignment with sales goals.

Step 1: The Business Objectives

- Clearly define the business objectives that sales and marketing strategies are supporting.
- Ensure they are clear and that everyone understands them.

Step 2: The Target Market

- Conduct a "patient segmentation" session. Consider the perspectives of both sales and marketing. By separating your teams (or separating your thinking), you will find differences that need to be overcome.
  - Talk about demographic profiles, purchasing behavior, needs, values, culture, and habits.

Step 3: The Definition of the Solution

- Define the solution your offering and what is desired by the patients. Then you can define a range of services to offer. Ask yourself the following questions:
  - What does your patient want?
  - How can you offer a solution?
  - What product or service should you be offering the patient?

Step 4: Gain a Strategic Position and Find a Unique Selling Proposition

- Analyze the key brand values and desired patient outcomes by asking the following questions:
  - What is the price patients are willing to pay?

- ◦ Do they require a quick turnaround?
- ◦ Do they need high-quality products and service?
- Use this information to define the position that your company should occupy within the marketplace.
  - ◦ Perform a competitor overview by comparing relative key strengths and weaknesses to identify opportunities. This review will lead to the definition of a unique selling proposition relative to other companies, which can be emphasized in marketing and sales activity.
- You are not just trying to market and sell to potential patients. You are trying to outmarket and outsell your competitors. This helps to align marketing and sales goals.

Step 5: Identify Marketing Objectives and Align Them With Sales Objectives

- Based on the business objectives, patient segmentation/value, and percentage of repeat business, you can start to model the number of new clients and patient retention rate required to achieve the revenue objectives.
- Some markets and some patients can be too expensive to acquire and maintain. It may require changing directions.

Step 6: Marketing Strategy

- Start with broad strategic frameworks including the following:
  - ◦ The identification of key marketing channels
  - ◦ The objective behind their use
  - ◦ The integration between channels
- Channels will include online communications such as social media, search engine organization, and email; sponsorships; event planning; and traditional advertising using direct mail, billboards, television, and print.
- Focus on each channel uniquely and then work out smart ways to integrate the ideas between channels.
- Maintain a cohesive message.

Step 7: Marketing Plan and Campaign Development

- Once you identify the strategy, you develop your marketing plan. Your plan should align with sales activities and the overall business objectives. It is one piece of the giant puzzle. The following are some tips for how you can break down the sales/marketing barrier within your own organization:
  - ○ Align the goals: Understanding revenue and content goals can provide a greater understanding of what the 2 teams are ultimately working toward. Your entire team should be aware of what drives revenue. Encourage members of your marketing team to sit in on sales calls and meetings. Your marketers can gather tremendous insight as to what messages resonate with your patients as well as the issues that may reduce sales. The sales team's unique perspective can be really valuable to the marketing team.
  - ○ Prioritize messaging: Creative marketing team members can be pulled in many different directions. Having someone from the sales side help to organize requests can build trust and increase efficiency. Set up regular meetings, giving both the sales and marketing team an opportunity to talk about current projects, future plans, and any obstacles that need to be addressed.
  - ○ Pipeline + revenue = alignment: The marketing team should feel accountable to sales not just for deliverables but also for measurable results. By demonstrating its commitment in terms of revenue, marketing will share the sales team's number one goal. This is the ultimate alignment.
  - ○ Optimize investments: Marketing has come to depend on detailed data and analytics to determine how and where to invest in digital channels, but when it comes to sales channels, marketing has little to no data about what content is helping sales close deals. Marketing members needs to understand which content is used by sales and, most importantly, which content is tied to closed revenue. With these insights, the marketing department can invest more in the content that affects revenue. The same insights give the sales team confidence in the content marketing is producing.
  - ○ People buy experiences; give them one: Our experiences and expectations as consumers are changing our behavior. Patients self-educate and want information on demand. More importantly, potential patients want to interact with sales only when necessary. Most sales teams have not adapted to changing patient expectations, and many marketers

do not focus on how they can improve interactions between sales and patients. Marketing should work with sales to provide content-driven solutions that empower sales members to do a guided sell when they are talking with a patient. Focusing on the patient and the patient's experience is a great way to align sales and marketing.

○ Culture: In addition to focusing on revenue, analytics, the patient, and the patient's experience, it is important to build a culture of collaboration. Agree to be objective. Learn to lean on each other and support one another. Most importantly, discuss the losses to improve, but always celebrate the wins.

CONCLUSION

Aligning your marketing and sales strategy may seem like a daunting task, but if you have the 2 teams successfully in place, it really comes down to creating a strong communication pipeline. Most leaders understand the need for this integration in theory but struggle to put it into practice.

Forming strong communication is a dance, a somewhat awkward dance to begin with, but with direct leadership and guidance, you will begin to see and feel synergy between the 2 teams. As a leader, you can often feel the need for control, but this mostly comes from ego. Creating a strong communication pipeline requires an element of trust and "letting go." To be successful, you must allow the marketing and sales teams to find their feet even though you have choreographed the steps.

REFERENCE

1.   Lewis ESE. Catch-line and argument. *The Book-Keeper*. 1903;15:124-128.

Section III

Tools Used in Marketing

Traditional Marketing

Michael Malley, BA and Jeremy Westby

Traditional marketing is a term commonly used today to describe the advertising methods employed before the evolution of online- and mobile-based marketing. This would include affiliate and cable network television advertising, print media (newspapers, magazines, and direct mail), radio advertising, and outdoor billboards, which have been a primary tool for advertising and marketing for decades.

As traditional as these media partners might seem in today's world of digital, broadband, and cellular marketing, a significant percentage of the ophthalmic marketing target audience (men and women 21 to 70 years of age) still watch local television programming, tune into their favorite radio stations, and drive by countless digital and printed billboards on their daily commutes. Although traditional newspaper and magazine readership has dropped significantly, online readership of digital versions of these publications has helped stabilize the loss.

One of the key challenges marketers have today with traditional media is the inability to use analytics to evaluate TV, radio, and print media performance.

Wang M, ed. *Grow Your Eye Care Practice:*
High-Impact Pearls From the Marketing Experts (pp 67-71).

Traditional media can deliver the number of estimated viewers, listeners, and readers they have, but they have little hard data to support their costs. That is why today's cable providers, affiliate television stations, radio stations, newspapers, and magazines are offering digital packages to supplement traditional methods. With traditional television advertising, stations now offer advertising access to streaming programming and video on demand where viewers can only view programming after watching a paid advertisement.

To supplement the lack of actual listenership analytics, radio stations are now offering marketers access to their listeners via email marketing and event marketing. They can also coordinate the precise run times of advertising messages with a correlating increase or decrease of website and landing page traffic to measure the overall effect of your messaging. To do this, stations need approval from the practice to access the back end of websites. Radio can also encompass podcasts, streaming, and voice-activated devices.

With each of the traditional marketing media partners, practices can use "earned media" (eg, interviews and other editorial coverage) to gain exposure and build brand without having to pay for the space. These are short-lived pieces but can provide a great return on your time invested. Press clippings can be used digitally or in print in subsequent advertising and brochures. The interviews can also be used in your social and digital marketing efforts and help bolster your reputation and validity in the marketplace.

To best incorporate traditional media, you must know your market and your competition. Identify your buyer's persona. Who do you want to reach with your message? If your target audience is in their 20s to 30s, you should take a hard look at digital media. Most millennials and Generation Xers are not actively using traditional media. They want their information quick, on demand, and brief. If you cannot get a billboard message, social ad, or commercial to them in 15 seconds or less, you are at risk of losing their attention.

Local advertising and marketing agencies have local, regional, and sometimes national marketing data. They also have tested capabilities to target demographic data and narrow your results to the outlets that are most effective, exposing your message to those who would be most likely (1) to make the decision to read about your product offering and (2) to make a near-term purchase decision. In the digital space, you can even select to advertise toward those potential customers who have already looked at ads served up by the competition.

The second step is to identify the most cost-effective methods for advertising. Although many advertisers would steer you in the direction of social and digital only, traditional media should not be overlooked. When properly used and leveraged, traditional media can deliver cost-effective results. Practices need to research which outlets in the traditional space best fit their budget and combine that with a mix of their social and digital media partners.

The third step centers on creating effective messages that are impactful, appealing, and contain a strong call to action. Because of the cost of today's marketing, it is imperative to quickly determine which one of your creative ads are performing best. This can be accomplished through a technique known as *split testing* or *A/B testing* in which you maintain the same media frequency and spending, changing *only* the message or design. By keeping all other variables the same, this technique allows the marketer to evaluate the performance of one message against the other. Continual testing of this type helps insure proper creative messaging and design are always in place.

One of the more effective ways to use traditional marketing is with the use of a spokesperson. Today, this is referred to as an *influencer* because of his or her potential to influence the public with his or her endorsement. In ophthalmic marketing, spokespersons and influencers are open to trading out their fees in exchange for refractive surgery. Be certain to negotiate a contract with the spokesperson based on him or her first working off the full amount of the refractive procedure he or she is receiving. Be sure to check with your state medical board for the specific regulations regarding patient testimonials. Be sure to have patients, spokespersons, and influencers sign at least 1-year contracts that give your practice the full rights and usage of their image and statements for traditional, social, and digital media. Understand that an influencer's reputation is highly scrutinized. One bad move by him or her can have a negative effect on your practice's reputation.

Television (broadcast and cable) advertising is a highly efficient, consistent performer to drive brand awareness to motivate and engage consumers. It is best suited for reaching broad anonymous audiences across a wide area. There is a perceived accountability with well-accepted audience measurement metrics. Television is relatively easy to buy with little maintenance after buying. It has a proven success record for promoting mass consumer products. Commercials attached to a well-researched media buying plan, based on accurate market data, can maximize your advertising dollar. However, there are disadvantages. The prime metric for traditional TV, gross ratings points, is based on an estimation. Advertisers have no way of knowing whether the people who are theoretically exposed to your ad during such programming actually saw it, and you will not know much about them except for their age and demographic. Increased video on demand and digital video recording use diminishes commercial effect. Many television shows skew to audiences of an older age and lower income. Prime time is no longer a preeminent reach builder. A large part of the viewing population is not substantially reached by prime-time networks. There is increased ad clutter in linear programming as the commercial pods lengthen. TV viewing is now possible over many devices, applications, and networks. Beyond traditional linear television advertising, you can access 100+ million households across national, local, video on demand, and addressable TV inventory. Less than one-third (28%) of brands have integrated digital audience data into their TV ad buys, although 68% plan to do so in the next 12 months.[1]

Radio (terrestrial and internet) listeners are loyal. Driven largely by an increase in the length of consumer commutes, the number of people listening to the radio has grown exponentially over the last decade. Research shows that radio still holds one of the highest return on investments in the industry. Media planners have access to research that will show what your customers listen to and when they listen. Use that data to your advantage. The downsides to radio include the ability to change stations quickly, causing fragmentation over multiple stations and formats. Satellite radio, streaming, and downloads have stolen significant audience share from radio stations. Recent acquisitions like SiriusXM, Pandora, and iHeartRadio (formerly Clear Channel; iHeartMedia, Inc) have provided partnerships to help bridge the gap between traditional and satellite broadcasts and the mobile user. There are many options to reach those users beyond a traditional radio buy. Advantages to radio advertising include the ability to target a demographic group with less expense, frequent messaging opportunities, and community appeal. Disadvantages include a lack of visual media, multiple stations and formats are required to accumulate message reach, and peak timing is typically during the morning and later afternoon commute while other times suffer a lower audience.

Billboards are located on key highways, intersections, and integral choke points throughout the country. Modern billboards include traditional static bulletins (print), digital, and trivisions (rotating vertical triangles). Digital bulletins add an extra layer of timeliness and relevance to your campaign, with creative messaging presented based on the time of day, weather, sports scores, or other unique information. A billboard should have no more than 7 words, the fewer the better. These ads should be big, bold, and believable. Research shows that when outdoor media is added to the overall plan, it increases the search return on advertising dollars spent by 40%[2] and drives 4 times more social/digital activations per ad dollar spent.[3] Consumers are 48% more likely to engage with a mobile ad after being exposed to the same ad on outdoor media.[4]

Print marketing includes newspapers, magazines, and direct mail. It has a touchy-feely effect because your messaging can be held, mulled over, and shared. Direct mail, display ads, coupons, magazine ads, advertorials, business cards, flyers, and sell sheets are easily created. With little distractions and no scrolling, print offers tangible reach to consumers. There are many options for advertising in the local daily and weekly papers. Each company should have rate cards readily available. Newspapers are one of the most expensive methods to reach your audience, with some charging as much as $25 for every 1000 who might see a half-page ad. Note that nearly 30% of newspaper reading is performed online.[5]

Direct mail remains the most expensive marketing method available. Interestingly, one study found direct mail takes 21% less cognitive effort to understand promotional material compared with online marketing.[6] With proper targeting, a printed messaging piece can be delivered into the hands of potential customers.

Although not normally considered traditional, bulk text messages (SMS) and autodialers are another way to market directly to potential customers. While large call centers would have banks of personnel cold-calling to generate leads, data companies can now provide geographic- and demographic-targeted lists to connect your brand to potential customers. This method should be narrowly targeted at consumers who have already expressed interest in your product.

REFERENCES

1. TVA Media Group. TV advertising isn't dead—it's evolving. Published March 2, 2019. Accessed August 4, 2020. https://www.tvamediagroup.com/tv-advertising-isnt-dead-its-evolving/

2. Out of Home Advertising Association of America. New study: out of home advertising delivers $5.97 in revenue ROI. Published May 16, 2017. Accessed August 24, 2019. https://oaaa.org/Portals/0/Public%20PDFs/2019%20-%20OOH%20By%20The%20Numbers.pdf?ver=2020-03-11-142451-873

3. Xaxis: The Outcome Media Company. Digital out of home: realizing the potential. Your guide to the programmatic DOOH opportunity and best practices to get started. Accessed August 4, 2020. https://www.xaxis.com/de/wp-content/uploads/2019/07/DOOH-Realizing-the-Potential-Xaxis-Whitepaper-2019.pdf

4. Traditional OOH and OUTFRONT mobile—a powerhouse duo. Out Front Media. Accessed October 28, 2019. https://www.outfrontmedia.com/media/mobile

5. Out of Home Advertising Association of America. Media comparison: what are the advantages and disadvantages of the major media formats? How does OOH complement them? Why is OOH advertising a good choice? Accessed August 4, 2020. https://oaaa.org/ProofOOHWorks/SalesTools/MediaComparison.aspx

6. Dopson E. Direct mail marketing: does it still work in 2019? Published March 29, 2018. Accessed August 4, 2020. https://www.lucidpress.com/blog/direct-mail-marketing-does-it-still-work

Marketing Using Social Media

John Mickner, BA

Small businesses lack the resources to compete with franchises and large corporate chains. For this reason, they often rely on a combination of retaining current customers and word-of-mouth marketing. In the past, these strategies were adequate to keep the business afloat or even prosper. Today, these strategies still work, but additional marketing methods must be added to be competitive. Although the focus of this book is directed toward professionals in the vision and eye care disciplines, the principles being laid out here can help professionals in any discipline or industry. The previously mentioned strategies of customer retention and word-of-mouth marketing worked well when you were the only game in town or the nearest competitor was in the next town or even farther away. Today, with mergers and acquisitions, franchising, and even organic expansion by big corporations, competition has not only exponentially increased, but it also can be stifling to the growth of your business.

On the daily commute to your office, it is not uncommon to see digital billboards and advertising wraps on buses or hear radio ads by competitors near

Wang M, ed. *Grow Your Eye Care Practice:*
High-Impact Pearls From the Marketing Experts (pp 73-77).
© 2021 Taylor & Francis Group.

your business location. Recently, I saw a large billboard perched on top of a 6-story building that advertised the same medical services as my friend who has an office several hundred feet away. This particular company is relatively new to the area but has the advertising power and budget of a billion-dollar national franchise. The billboard was so large that it was impossible to miss. The ad stated that the practice was the best in the area with the most competitive prices. My heart sank for a minute as I empathized with my friend who must pass this billboard on a daily basis. What resonated with me was the thought that not only was the enemy at the gates but also that the enemy is virtually in my friend's waiting room. What can my friend do to compete with this big corporate competitor?

The good news is that in today's digital marketing age, small practices like my friend's can go on the counterattack on multiple fronts and within budget. There are social media tools available to small business that can help to retain patients, encourage word-of-mouth testimonials, and garner referrals. Social media can be done for free or very little cost, whereas the traditional marketing methods can be extremely expensive and involve contract commitments. Usually, the only way to get substantial discounts using traditional methods is to enter into a long-term contact. If they do not get the intended results, it can become a poor investment.

Although social media marketing may not cost you money directly, you must pay someone to create the media. Someone must maintain an effective campaign. An employee may be assigned this additional task, but be careful that it is someone who enjoys it and will take it on as a welcome assignment. An employee with marketing experience or social media savvy is preferred. If you do not have an employee who meets these criteria, consider hiring someone who does. Options include a young person from a local high school or a college student who is eager to work and willing to be paid an entry-level pay rate. Look for a high school or college that has a curriculum that includes some type of information technology or computer skills program. Most young folks today are social media savvy. Consider students who will do this as part of an apprenticeship program. They get course credits, and you might not have to pay any wages at all. Whoever you assign to this task must understand how critical social media marketing is to the life of your business. You should offer incentives for good work and proven results.

There are many ways to track results using the various social media applications and platforms. In my opinion, social media enables businesses to track marketing results more effectively and accurately than traditional methods at a fraction of the cost. Additionally, most results from social media marketing can be determined in a much shorter time period than traditional methods. This allows business owners to be more agile in marketing and make adjustments to marketing methods and campaign strategies more quickly with less stress. You can even get your staff and patients involved as part of your social media campaigns and give them their moment of recognition.

BRANDING IS VITAL

Branding is the process of creating a name, logo, symbol, and personality to represent your product or service. Brands become valuable when customers associate high value and quality products or services with a product. Branding creates a memorable imprint on consumers' brains that helps establish awareness and long-term loyalty. It provides a consistent image so consumers know what to expect. Satisfaction is based on meeting or exceeding expectations.

Base your brand identity on the product or service's key value proposition, which is the number one reason why consumers would engage you. The proposition should be stated in a clear, succinct manner across all social media. Base all future communications on this image.

Part of a brand identity involves the visual representation of it, which includes the logo, colors, type font, and other design aspects. Keep color consistent throughout your web page and any social media you use. The font and logos can create a great deal of emotion. The most important thing is readability and accessibility. Creativity can lead to pretty, artistic fonts, but these are not as easy to read. Again, be consistent across all websites and social media postings.

CREATE BRAND AWARENESS

Once you have your brand's value proposition and image, you can use your website and social media to build awareness. Investigate your target market to determine where they are located, what sites they frequent online, and what influencers they follow.

Start producing content on your sites as well as external sites that your target market might read. Produce as much different content as possible, and keep it current to provide value to your customer. Give readers a reason to come back and learn more. Do this at least on a weekly basis.

Businesses that blog regularly get 97% more inbound business. Give your blog a unique name. Link to as many other social media channels that you can.

Make it easy for other people to share or link to your material by using linking buttons. Press releases are especially useful and can increase your search ranking with Google. Post online videos and podcasts. The more you saturate the internet, the more likely the customer can find your product. As you continue to build your social media presence, do not change your brand. Do not change the logo, slogan, or any part of your brand identity. Keep your customers engaged long term. Keep your conversations active and current so that customers want to participate in your communication efforts continually.

Give customers rewards to bring more customers to you. Promote your product by encouraging happy patients to rate your services and provide feedback online. There are many ways to create customer loyalty programs using giveaways for attending informational seminars and bringing guests. Social media sites are the most effective way to promote these events. More information on increasing referrals and customer loyalty programs will be addressed within this textbook.

How Do I Get People to Find My Website?

The short answer is search engine optimization. Using search engine optimization techniques will increase traffic to your website by catering to Google's formula. Pull together a few different keywords or phrases that speak to your content. Sprinkle them throughout your title, meta descriptions and tags, and content if you so desire. Try to imagine what people type into the search bar to find your website on Google and adjust accordingly. When people find your website, they will also see your social media link buttons.

Word of Mouth

Tell your friends and family about your website and social media sites. Invite them to "like" your Facebook page and "follow" you on Facebook, Instagram, Twitter, and LinkedIn. Your contacts can help spread your URL and social media sites. Investigate local media contests where you can have patients and friends vote for your practice. Consider local media where businesses may be spotlighted and see how to be listed. Assuming you win or receive recognition as being one of the best in your profession or industry in your area, you can use that good press to post on all your social media sites. Ask all of your social media contacts to post this news on their sites. One article that I posted on Twitter about a year ago was liked by several people who then retweeted the article to their contacts. I was astounded to find out that it reached 23,000 people.

Promote your social media sites on your website with links on one or more pages. Request patients and friends visit your website and social media sites. If your friends have their phones handy, ask them to go to your site or sites and see the latest updates while you wait for a train or dinner.

Make sure your business cards include your social media information. Your most important calling cards are your business card, website, and social media sites. Millennials, in particular, will look at social media first in order to research companies, products, or services in which they are interested. They buy electronics and cars, schedule vacations, and book appointments for all types of medical care online. The more interesting and up to date your website and social media content is, the more likely they are to contact you for your services. Truth be told, if they cannot find you on social media, you will not see them at your practice.

In addition to having your own social media sites, you should join industry-related social media groups if possible. Join conversations and dialogues with group peers. This may not be seen by your patients or prospects, but it could lead to cross referrals from other group members.

ADVERTISING ON SOCIAL MEDIA

I am not a big proponent of paid ads on social media, but further investigation will determine if this would be good in your particular area. People do respond very well to giveaways, promotions, deals, and free resources or items. Offering something to your users attracts more of them. Attract the right audience through "brand ambassadors." A brand ambassador program can be used to attract more of the same followers and customers to accomplish your goal. Many users are willing to be brand ambassadors for a small discount or deal, so you will not spend any extra money on marketing.

11

Websites, Search Engine Optimization, and Online Consultation

Michael Weiss, BS, MBA

To a modern eye care practice, a website is a critical necessity for long-term success. An eye care provider should communicate the professionalism of his or her practice through the website. It will be the first interaction many patients have with the practice's brand. As such, focusing on having a high-quality website should be a top priority within the overall marketing strategy. This section covers several topics on websites. The first issue covered is why esthetic design is an important complement to functionality and structure. Key concepts are then discussed including writing content, responsive website design, Americans With Disabilities Act (ADA) compliance, navigation, and other important terminology. Finally, content management systems, website security, and how to measure the effectiveness of a website are explained.

Wang M, ed. *Grow Your Eye Care Practice:*
High-Impact Pearls From the Marketing Experts (pp 79-103).

DESIGN AND PATIENT EXPERIENCE

A well-designed visual layout and appearance of an eye care provider's website will help educate potential new patients more effectively by letting them find answers to their questions more quickly. It will also be effective for converting new website visitors into patients. Furthermore, many patients will be impressed by a design that adopts modern standards. These standards include easy readability, allowing users to quickly find the desired information they seek. A recent study showed that the most commonly agreed-on critical elements for a website design were logical organization, content relevance and usefulness, navigation, well-used multimedia content such as contrasting colors, and an immediate clear statement of the purpose of the website.[1] By successfully addressing and incorporating these items into the design and visual layout, the website will be a more effective marketing tool.

A strong website design will strengthen the appeal of the website and ultimately lead to new patients. Studies have indicated that one's emotional experience is connected to one's perception of how well it works, so the sheer esthetics of a website cannot be ignored. A Stanford University–based study that examined thousands of users found that although many other factors play a significant part, the professional look and feel of the website is by far the most important part to determine a website's credibility.[2] Although there is no right or wrong color theme or specific requirements, aiming for professionalism in the design is critical for maximizing the success of the website.

The following specific elements are necessary for a strong website design in order to help achieve practice goals and a positive patient interaction:

- Straightforward navigation menu
- Prominent contact information or contact forms
- Easy-to-locate provider credentials
- Coordinated color scheme
- Professional design that invokes the appropriate user emotions
- Balanced spacing and even margins
- Easy-to-read, legible fonts
- Functionality across all device types, especially mobile devices

The patient's interactive experience with the website should be positive. To create a frictionless website session, the physician and the website developer should avoid common sources of frustration. The following are several common pitfalls with websites that can hurt the patient experience:

- Content is hard to find.
- Web pages load too slowly.
- Font sizes are too small to read.
- Short line height makes each line too close together.
- Large image files prevent the page from loading.
- Key components, like the main navigation, do not function properly.
- The mobile phone experience is poor or confusing.
- ADA compliance, which has recently seen an increase in enforcement in 2018,[3] is lacking.
- A missing call to action prevents patients from contacting the office.
- Website security is compromised.

These drawbacks are very common. It is estimated that less than 50% of all websites have code that will pass a validation check based on published aggregated data submitted to an online validation checker.[4] A high price tag for the development of a website does not guarantee that it will be free of these problems. Some of these drawbacks have very measurable and immediate negative effects. For example, if users find themselves waiting over 5 seconds for a website to load, the probability that the user will leave more than doubles.[5] This means that the potential new patient may then return to Google and end up find a competing website. If the website loads, but it is unclear how to contact the office, the patient may not contact the office at all. Because of the complexity of modern website design, even after launch, regular testing and/or monitoring is necessary to ensure that websites remain functional.

A Responsive Website Design Is a Necessity

A responsive website design will dynamically adapt the display, layout, and functionality of the website to the device being used. For example, the content will adapt and display optimally for a phone, tablet, or desktop. Many responsive websites will adapt to up to 4 different devices' size configurations, such as a desktop, notebook computer, tablet, or smartphone. This type of dynamic development is critical for an effective website, but it will require additional work from the website developer.

A common problem when designing a website is paying too much attention to the desktop version. This can happen because correspondence with the website developer and physician is still conducted via email, phone, desktop, or laptop computers. However, mobile traffic climbed from less than 1% of traffic in 2009 to over 50% of all website traffic in 2018.[6] A study from Google has shown that these mobile visitors have rapidly increased the rate in which they convert from a visitor to a customer.[7] Because these mobile visitors are such a high priority, many websites are being designed with a "mobile first" framework that has the website developer design the website keeping the mobile experience in mind first and then adapting the resulting website to desktop views. Providers should focus on building a responsive website and focus especially on the mobile interaction experience.

COMMON WEBSITE COMPONENTS AND TERMINOLOGY

When an eye care provider engages a firm to develop a website, it can be useful to understand the common website layout sections and related common terminology specific to website design. A few common terms are outlined for reference:

- Domain name: The domain name of the website ends in a .com, .org, etc and is in each part of the name. The most commonly used extension for commercial websites is .com.
- URL: The URL is the address of a page that is typed into the website address bar. Each URL will always have a domain name followed by a slash (/) and the label for the specific page, which is sometimes called a *slug*.
- Page: A website consists of a set of individual pages, each with their own URL.
- Website host: When visitors view a website page, they are seeing information that exists on another remote or virtual computer.
- Header: The header of the website is the upper portion that is generally the same across all pages of the website. It will usually include a horizontal navigation bar that is below or above it. The header will include the logo, social media icons, contact information, or important links.
- Navigation: The main navigation is the set of structured links to the important pages of the website. The navigation is generally always accessible.

- Main content section: Each page has a main section that contains the content on the page. It can be divided into different sections and sometimes contains a sidebar with additional navigational items, contact forms, or information relevant to the specific website page.
- Footer: The footer of the page is the final component of the website that sits on the bottom of the page. The footer, like the header, should be standardized for all pages of the website.
- HTML: This is the programming language used by website developers to encode the website pages' structure and content. It consists of wrapping different parts of the website in tags.
- Tag: An HTML tag is the fundamental building block for websites. Tags are nested in a hierarchical structure. Each tag is used to define either a container of content or an individual part of the content such as an image, link, heading, or figures.
- CSS: The programming language used to visually style the HTML code to add colors, margins, fonts, background images, and responsive functionality.
- JavaScript: The programming language used by website developers to add all functionality to the website beyond the content and its styling such as tracking.
- Plug-in: A website plug-in is an existing utility that a website developer can include on the website to perform a needed function. The plug-in significantly reduces development time.

WEBSITE NAVIGATION

Navigation of the website is one of the most essential aspects of its design. Navigation of the website must be consistent across all pages. Having consistent navigation makes it easier for visitors to find what they are looking for as they browse across different pages of the website. If the main navigation changes for certain pages or sections of the website, it will be especially confusing for patients. A modern feature of navigation is to have an anchored navigation that is accessible from the header of the website, even as the user scrolls down the page. An example of a website desktop navigation is shown in Figure 11-1. It is also important to format websites for mobile devices and tablets. The same menu has been dynamically adjusted to display on a mobile site in Figure 11-2.

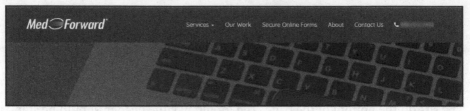

Figure 11-1. An example of website desktop navigation.

Figure 11-2. Adaptation of the desktop navigation for use on mobile devices is critical. This is an example of the navigation in Figure 11-1 formatted for a mobile phone.

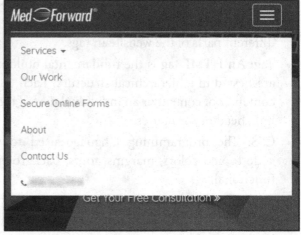

Figure 11-3. When creating a website, breadcrumbs are used to show how the user reached a certain page and how to access the parent pages.

About LASIK
Treatments » Laser Procedures » LASIK

There is no fixed rule for the amount of links on a navigation menu. Offering fewer options is not necessarily better. Ideally, the navigation menu should be focused on what is the most logical and easily understandable for website visitors. The font size in the navigation menu should be large enough to be easily read.

"Breadcrumbs" are a set of a hierarchical links that show how the user reached a certain page and how to access the parent pages. For example, a set of breadcrumbs may appear similar to the one shown in Figure 11-3. Generally, each page on a website has a parent page, and the breadcrumbs let users quickly find their way back to that parent page.

The navigation menu can be customized for a website's logical content organization but, at a minimum, needs to include links to the following resources:

- An about us page that includes biographies of the eye care providers
- A contact information page with the phone numbers, contact form, location, and office hours
- A procedure page or pages that provide an overview of the procedures with links to each of the procedure pages

A home page link can be included in the main navigation but does not have to be present if the logo is placed in the header in such a location that clicking on it can be used to return to the home page.

The order of the elements in the navigation menu should include the links of greatest importance to the left because visitors click left to right. In the case of a vertically stacked menu, it should read from top to bottom in the order of importance. The exception to this rule is the contact information link that can be placed in the rightmost position, which is the common placement.[8] It is also acceptable to place a contact information link as a prominent button above the navigation bar in the header.

COMPLIANCE WITH THE AMERICANS WITH DISABILITIES ACT WEBSITE REQUIREMENTS

Compliance with the regulations under the ADA helps improve a website's search engine optimization (SEO), makes a website easier to interact with for all users, and makes it possible for users with disabilities to still use the website.[9] Although there are third-party software tools that a website developer can quickly install to help with ADA compliance, installing this tool by itself is not enough to ensure compliance. Many of the components of ADA compliance overlap with the best practices already in place with website design, but some of them are subtler and could be overlooked. The following are some of the most important ADA compliance steps, but by no means are they inclusive of all requirements[10-12]:

- The website should be easy to navigate with a consistent means of navigation across the entire website.
- A user should be able to hit the "Tab" button on the keyboard to navigate all website links on the website, including the main navigation.
- All images need to have alternate text that accurately provides a very brief description of the image for visually impaired users.

- Images should not contain text unless that text is in a logo.
- Contact forms should have fields that are very clearly labeled.
- If a contact form has certain requirements, the instructions should be clear, and any invalid input error messages should clearly provide instructions on how to proceed.
- If the website has a video, there should be an option to view the transcription of the video.
- The use of "Click Here" or "Read More" as link text should be avoided. Instead, make the link describe the target page.
- The page title should make logical sense for every page.
- A form cannot rely on a user to press "Enter" without providing a button to perform the same function. The form needs to have a corresponding well-labeled action button. Examples of appropriately named action buttons include "Search" or "Send Email" next to the input fields on a search form or contact us via email form, respectively.
- Each page needs to have one primary heading that identifies what the page is about to website users. Website developers must use a specific HTML tag known as the H1 tag to encode this heading. This tag should be used only once per page.

WEBSITE CONTENT AND COMPONENTS

Online Contact Form

An online contact form is a crucial element for getting the best results from a website. Many times, website visitors may not be browsing the website during a provider's main business hours when phone lines are open, or, alternatively, they may be unable to call. If the website contains an online form, these potential new patients can fill out an online contact request and begin the conversation. This type of nonphone contact method applies to website visitors of all ages and is especially important for attracting younger patients who are more accustomed to text message communications.[13]

Email Marketing Sign-Up Form

Email marketing is an important component of a modern online marketing strategy. In addition to collecting email addresses from existing patients at the office, placing an easy-to-use online newsletter sign-up form on the website will allow for a larger base of interested visitors to receive email communications.

Writing Content for the Website

For the physician creating a new website, creating content for the website may seem like a daunting task. Although writing the content can involve a significant commitment of one's time, it is important to make this task a high priority within the marketing strategy. The quality of the website content is closely linked with SEO.

An important first step is to create an outline for the website. The outline should include, at a minimum, a home page, a page for each procedure and physician, and a patient resources page that covers issues such as insurance information and answers to commonly asked administrative questions.

After the initial outline is completed, providers should prepare content for the home page (which will be the most frequently visited page) as well as a page for each procedure. For SEO, it is important to include at least 300 words per page, including the home page. Sometimes the trend is to have a minimal home page design in a modern website, but it still should include at least 300 words. Providing educational content to patients is important. Internet users are becoming increasingly interested in educating themselves by searching online.[14]

The website should include, if possible, a testimonial page that highlights patient success stories or positive real online reviews. However, it is important to check state or federal laws and regulations to determine what is allowed in this type of marketing. The laws may vary for each state. Also, some professional medical organizations or licensing boards may restrict what type of patient testimonial writing is permitted. The website should include a "results may vary for each patient" statement on the footer of the page so that Google will approve algorithmically of this type of content.

If a single page on the website is overly complex, excessively lengthy, or packed with too many images, it may hurt the effectiveness of the page.[15] To fix this, divide complex pages into separate pages and avoid overlapping material. A good philosophy is to aim for the best possible patient experience.

Keep Website Content Up to Date

Website content absolutely needs to stay current and up to date. Even after the website is constructed, eye care providers should schedule a recurring task to review the website for any needed changes. Patients may not have a good first impression of the practice if there is clearly outdated information present on the website. Also, because the practice website is a critical patient communication tool, there is a huge marketing opportunity cost associated with not posting information about new procedures to the website.

Common Pitfalls for Website Content Writing

Missing the Target Audience

Because physicians are highly trained and experienced in their field, their writing may be at an advanced level that is out of reach of the target audience for the website. On a daily basis, a physician's writing will include medical patient encounter notes for either him- or herself or other doctors. Furthermore, if the physician contributes to professional journals, the research writing will be highly sophisticated and intended for advanced audiences. Continuing medical education courses and material that physicians read on a regular basis will also be at this advanced level. Because of the reading and writing that eye care providers work with on a regular basis, what comes naturally to them may not be suitable for the patients reading the information on the website.

When preparing the information, make sure to use terms and sentences that laypeople can understand and easily process. It may help to have someone else read the information and provide feedback, help adjust the tone, or even complete the writing of the content that the eye care provider outlines for him or her.

Not Being Direct and to the Point

Website visitors expect to be able to start reading about the information being presented in the heading of a page right away. Sometimes, physicians provide too much historical context around a procedure or related information that does not directly address the procedure for that specific page of the website. It is best to ensure that the content is direct and to the point in discussing the topic a patient came to that page to find.

CONTENT MANAGEMENT SYSTEMS AND WEBSITE PLATFORMS

Websites can be developed with pure code, or they can use a content management system. There are benefits and drawbacks to each approach. For example, a content management system empowers eye care providers to be able to update content themselves without a website developer, but they also require regular software updates and more expensive website hosting.

Overview of Platforms

No Platform Approach

The no platform approach uses pure code. If coded well and efficiently, the no platform method can involve lower hosting fees, faster website performance, and a higher level of security. The primary drawbacks are that every update will require the involvement of a website developer and could be more expensive.

Open-Source Free Platforms

The are several popular open-source free content management systems that can be used as a platform for a website. The 3 content management systems that collectively have the largest market share include Joomla (Open Source Matters, Inc), Drupal, and WordPress (Automattic).

WordPress[16] currently has the largest market share of all platforms at over 60%. The sheer popularity of the WordPress platform has made it a standard. Because of its widespread use, many plug-ins are available to help add new features and functionality to a website. One advantage of this platform is that physicians can more easily switch between website development companies because the platform has widespread adoption and support from multiple companies. It began as a blogging tool and thus makes adding a blog article or other project more cost effective than having this performed by an outside firm each time.

If a content management system is configured incorrectly or is using an out-of-date prebuilt theme or template, this can make the website slow, less robust, and subject to security vulnerabilities. Furthermore, it is important that content management is configured such that content updates made by those who are not website developers still have a consistent professional layout.

Proprietary Platforms

Some website companies offer their own content management system or proprietary platform as part of a marketing package. These can work very well, but they may come at a higher price, and it may be harder to later switch to another company. It is important to evaluate their abilities, past results, and functionalities carefully before committing to a proprietary system.

HOSTING, ENCRYPTION, AND SECURITY

Having a website that loads very quickly is pivotal in getting the best possible investment return. Larger firms like Google have studied the effect of a slow loading time on their websites.[17] For each fraction of a second after a page has been loaded, they have proved that a certain percentage of visitors will give up. This translates into a direct loss of revenue for a medical practice. Although the coding of the website and the images can be a factor, using a fast website server is very important. Content management systems will require extra computing resources and special features to run quickly. Likewise, having a secure server is paramount. The website host should include a real-time security monitoring and virus detection tool. The frequency of cyberattacks is increasing with each year.[18] Adding a secure certificate to the website, although it does not guarantee website security or Health Insurance Portability and Accountability Act (HIPAA) compliance by itself, is an added measure of security that is highly recommended. The certificate helps visitors ensure the website is authentic, encrypts all data between the visitor and the website, and adds the "https://" prefix to the URL.

SELECTING A WEBSITE DEVELOPMENT COMPANY

To select good website developers or development companies, it is important to examine the quality of their work portfolio, find existing client references, and ensure that they are being honest with their assessments and recommendations. An eye care provider should be patient and examine existing work. It is important to ask the company who will own the rights to the work produced. By default, contractors may have intellectual property of their creations unless a contract states otherwise. If the website company's work or most recent projects meet the quality standards that have been outlined in this chapter, then the company may be a good fit.

It is also prudent that the proposal outlines as many project details as possible, including the number of web pages, the SEO services that will be performed, and a project timeline. Another important credential for the company is its coding ability. With the widespread prevalence of beginner website development tools, some website companies do not actually have anyone who knows how to code in HTML or CSS. Although companies may be able to produce a website, it is best to determine if they know how to code or if they are using tools to build the website. If the developer is relying on high-level tools that do not have the coding experience necessary to build a custom website, the quality, loading speed, SEO, functionality, longevity, and effectiveness of a website will suffer.

MEASURING A WEBSITE'S PERFORMANCE

Monitoring the performance of the website is a necessity for long-term success. By examining the traffic and leads from the website carefully, physicians can learn where adjustments need to be made to content or layout, find pages that may not be working well, identify problems quickly so they can be resolved, and determine which marketing campaigns are working.

There are several commonly used tools to measure website traffic. One common, popular, and powerful free tool is Google Analytics.[19] This tool, when installed on a website, gives providers powerful detailed reports about website traffic. Although the tool does not give specific personal identifying information about visitors, such as one's name or phone number, it does show how many people visit the website as well as other important visitor behaviors and trends. For example, it will show a breakdown of mobile device visitors vs desktop visitors. The tool can also indicate what percentage of traffic came from people conducting searches on Google. Google Analytics can also show how long visitors have spent on the website and which pages they visited.

The following are some important term definitions for understanding Google Analytics or any tool that is used to measure website performance:

- Bounce rate: The bounce rate measures the percentage of website visitors who visit a website but do not interact any further. Visitors that "bounce" do not click on anything or interact any further. There is no exact rule for what this percentage should be. Generally, a bounce is a negative measurement that should be as low as possible. It is not a perfect measurement because some users who appear to bounce have actually called the office and their bounce is positive. However, tracking a bounce rate over time to determine if a bounce rate suddenly increases can be useful to determine if there is a problem. Bounce rates can vary for each industry and source of website traffic and vary from 20% to 90% as the normal rate.[20]

- Hits: A website hit is a measurement of every time a website visitor loads a page on a website. For example, if the visitor views 5 pages on the website, it will count as 5 hits. Tools that measure traffic to a website will provide visitor traffic statistics that include hits but also the total number of visitors who can have multiple hits per visit.

- Conversion rate: A conversion means that a website visitor completed a marketing goal for the website such as filling out an online form, placing a phone call to the office, or visiting several important pages on the website. The conversion rate is the percentage of visitors who convert into active prospects by completing a conversion. Keeping careful track of conversions and conversion rates over time is helpful for online marketing campaigns so that their success and performance can be measured relative to one another. The target conversion rates can vary and should be specific to the marketing goal actions and type of marketing campaign.

- Direct traffic: Direct traffic to the website is from visitors who type the website address directly into the web browser and do not use a search engine at all. This traffic is useful to measure because it reflects general baseline interest in a practice as a result of all marketing sources combined.

- Organic traffic: The term *organic traffic* is used to refer to traffic that has come from nonpaid search engine searches such as Google or Bing. This measurement is useful in determining the effectiveness of SEO that boosts the organic traffic. Knowing the volume of organic traffic is important, but some key search terms are more valuable than others for practice growth. It is important to track both the amount of search traffic and the search terms being used to obtain that traffic.

Many of the website traffic reports include both bounce and conversion rate metrics. There are many factors that can influence bounce and conversion rates. If the website is too slow to load, the bounce rate will be too high. If the design is difficult for patients to navigate or not mobile friendly, the bounce rate will be high, and the conversion rate will be low. If the website design directs a user's focus to the wrong part of the page, it can lower a conversion rate as well.

There are other types of traffic analysis that can be used for analyzing the effectiveness of a website. For example, heat map analysis provides a visual display of where visitors are clicking on the website. Comparable to an infrared photograph overlaid on the webpage, areas are shaded on a color spectrum based on the mouse activity and clicks. Any areas that are attracting attention or missing attention can be identified. Additional tools outside of Google Analytics may be required to generate heat map analysis.

Another analysis tool is A/B testing. A/B testing may not always be necessary but can be useful in marketing scenarios in which larger budgets or high amounts of website traffic are involved. A/B testing allows eye care providers to try different ideas and configurations at the same time and measure the success of each approach.

SEARCH ENGINE OPTIMIZATION

A search engine's goal is to provide results that are relevant to users when they search for topics. They use a database of all websites to quickly provide a ranked list of results based on an algorithm. The algorithm takes into consideration many advanced factors including the location of the user, the type of device the user is using to search, links between different websites, web page content, and other advanced factors.[21] When a potential new patient types in his or her topic as a search query in Google, the important parts of that query are called *keywords*. For example, a keyword may be "LASIK," and a keyword phrase could be "LASIK in Detroit, MI."

After the algorithm quickly returns the list of results, the rank is where the eye care provider's website displays for a keyword or keyword phrase. Although being the first search result is the best, placing within the first 10 results on the first page is much better than falling to the second page. Depending on the terms, as many as 71% to 92% of users do not click to go to the second page of search results.[22] SEO is a challenging and complex task that focuses on helping websites rank as high as possible. In some cases, it may be a year from a new website launch before it starts ranking well on search engines. For existing websites, SEO improvements may take several months to take effect. SEO is more challenging in densely populated cities than in less populated areas.

Selection of Keywords

It is important not to completely rely on intuition for the selection of keywords. It is easier to optimize for keywords and search terms that people do not frequently use. Instead, a database of actual search terms should be consulted to determine the best search targets.

First, identify the procedures and terms that are important for the practice. For example, it could be a general term like *eye care* or *ophthalmologist* or a procedure-specific term such as *cataract surgery*. Google offers access to its database of search frequency by geographic area through a tool called the *keyword planner* available through its advertising platform Google Ads. This tool can be accessed for free to identify terms that will yield the most traffic. The advertising market value of these search terms for new visitors is displayed alongside the frequency of searches.

Some terms are more competitive than others. The highly competitive terms are much more challenging to optimize on websites because so many practices are targeting these same terms to boost their SEO. Eye care providers can optimize for longer but less frequently used and less competitive variants of highly competitive terms if they are having trouble ranking a new website.

SEARCH RESULTS AND THE ROLE OF METADATA

A single search engine result generally appears as follows:

The Title of the Page
https://www.domainname.com/full-page-url
A brief description of the page is included here that should provide visitors with a short summary of what is on the page and why they would like to visit it.

The search result consists of the title; the URL for the page; and then, below the URL, the page description. The website developer can suggest what Google uses for the title and description sections by encoding it in the HTML. The URL is completely determined by the website developer. The title will also appear in the tab of a web browser across the top of the screen above the URL, but it is not visible on the page itself. This information, in addition to being important for ADA compliance as previously discussed, is also highly important for SEO.

The keyword phrase should appear in the URL, description, and title at least once. It can be helpful to find examples of effective titles and descriptions. To do this, perform a search for a competitive term and examine the titles, URLs, and descriptions of the pages that appear first in the search results. Also, it is important to remember that Google will ignore a website's title and description if it is ineffective or inaccurate. There is no obligation from the search engine to use what the website provides.

This invisible information contained in the title and description is called *metadata*. However, there are other types of metadata in addition to the title and description. The other metadata of importance includes the headings on the pages, such as the main heading or H1, for each page. In addition, images need to be assigned descriptions for visually impaired users. This description is called *alternate text* (sometimes called *alt text* for short).

When adding a new page to the website such as a blog post or new procedure, it can be easy to forget to check the parts that are invisible such as the metadata. Make sure to still focus on these SEO-related properties.

Another factor in search results is buggy code. The website code could contain minor bugs that are invisible to users but still exist behind the scenes. Sometimes invalid code will still look acceptable, but it does not follow the rules of proper coding. A website developer should use a code validator to help identify and correct these issues.[23]

CONTENT GUIDELINES FOR
SEARCH ENGINE OPTIMIZATION

Adhering to the content guidelines and recommendations will provide a boost to SEO, but there are additional factors that can increase the SEO for the website. First, it is important to recognize that the search results return specific pages on a website. Therefore, the website should be organized so that pages are written to optimize for a term. Although it is possible to include multiple related terms on a specific page, it is less effective to develop 1 page that covers 2 unrelated keyword terms, such as 2 specific procedures. Modern SEO is extremely competitive, and if a page is not focused on the keyword topic, it will not rank well for it.

Because search engines try to provide results that are relevant to the users searching for the term, it is important to make sure the content itself is about the term. The keyword should be used as frequently as necessary but should not be overused on the page. Search engines will penalize for manipulations that they see as designed to be purely for SEO purposes, such as "keyword stuffing."[24]

In addition to making sure each page is focused on the content, it is also recommended to include a few geographic references, such as the name of the city that one is targeting with the content. This will help increase the likelihood of the website appearing in searches that contain the city's name.

Another strategy to boost SEO is to include a wide variety of media types on a page. The page should include strong text content; a video; one or more images; links to relevant external websites; or other types of resources, such as a patient handout with additional information.

BACKLINKS TO A WEBSITE

Another factor that search engines use in their algorithms for determining a rank is how many websites link to a website. More important and relevant websites will generally have many websites linking to it. However, not all these inbound links are equally important in boosting SEO. A link from a major reputable news organization would provide a higher value than a link from a website that no one visits.

These links can also be associated with keywords or subject matter. The ranking of specific keywords for an eye care provider's website may be increased based on the content of the website that is providing the backlink. For example, a link from a reputable website that provides patients with information about the LASIK procedure and recommended eye care providers would offer greater value than a friend's blog about city services.

Because backlinks provide a boost to SEO, some SEO techniques involve purchasing links to artificially boost ranking. Google has placed measures in effect to penalize rankings of sites that try to take this approach, so it is best to rely on genuine links. The negative approach is called *black hat SEO* and involves using tricks and deception. Years ago, there were many easy tricks a developer could deploy to artificially boost rankings. Over time, Google added detection methods to the algorithm and penalized for the vast majority of these tricks. Black hat SEO still exists and, if not detected by search engines, can be very effective to provide a boost to SEO. However, the methods used can be both unethical and risky for long-term positioning. For these reasons, legitimate white hat SEO is the only method recommended. White hat SEO includes all approaches that comply with Google's recommendations and policies. By focusing on providing the best website for patients with white hat SEO approaches, SEO goals can be achieved as part of a viable long-term strategy.

A public relations firm may be able to help providers gain additional media coverage; this can produce legitimate backlinks that in turn will boost SEO rankings. Registering a website with other organizations or useful directories will also provide helpful backlinks.

Furthermore, a website will slowly gain backlinks over time from various other websites across the internet. A website that has been around for a long time is more likely to rank well than a brand-new website that has received little publicity.

LOCAL OPTIMIZATION

Sometimes a business can appear under several different but similar names. These can confuse search engine rankings in certain cases. To prevent this, it is best to use a local SEO listing service to push the correct version of the name across different directories on the internet. This practice is sometimes referred to as *local SEO*.

PAGE SPEED

A fast and secure website will rank better on Google.[25] To improve the loading speed, the website developer should run the website through a page speed analysis tool and then optimize according to the recommendations. This may include optimizing all images on the website and including additional coding best practice to improve the website's performance. In addition to reducing the bounce rate, the website will ultimately perform better in the rankings.

ONLINE REVIEWS AND SOCIAL MEDIA

Search engines use online reviews to help determine the ranking of a website. The number of reviews that the website or business receives will affect the ranking. Moreover, the content of the reviews and specific words within the review will be used for ranking. For example, if an eye care provider's reviews frequently include the word "LASIK," this will help improve search rankings for the LASIK keyword.

Patients frequently will leave a review on Yelp, Google, Bing, or other popular listings. These companies offer eye care providers the ability to register their practice listing. It is very important for providers to complete this step with all possible listing companies. This enables providers to monitor reviews in real time. In addition, these tools will often let business owners upload photos of their business as well as add descriptions that contain keywords, categories, and other pertinent information that will affect SEO.

Having and maintaining an active social media presence will also contribute to a strong overall SEO strategy. Search engines may examine the subject matter and popularity of the social media posts. The power of social media as both a referral tool and an SEO tool should not be underestimated. Posts containing the keyword terms will help with SEO. It is also helpful if social media posts include a link back to the website periodically. Furthermore, for video sharing sites like YouTube, it can be helpful to include a link to the website in the video description as well as embedding the video directly on the website.

SEARCH ENGINE OPTIMIZATION TOOLS

It is important to be extremely careful with the use of automated online SEO tools. Some of these tools may use out-of-date methods to submit to certain directories that could be flagged by Google as paid links and hurt SEO. The better SEO tools to use include monitoring and optimization tools that can track search engine positions and assist with configuring the SEO settings that have been outlined. The following tools can be useful in an SEO strategy or may be used by a website development company:

- Moz: This tool monitors the performance of the website for terms and their search rank. Moz also has a local directory optimization tool that can create consistent listings across different directory services. This company can automatically identify issues on pages that can negatively affect SEO. The tool can also assist with optimizing specific pages for SEO terms.

- Yoast: If the website runs on WordPress, the Yoast plug-in will let a website manager edit titles and descriptions or identify potential SEO issues with pages. It offers quick links for each page to fix page validations or other problems. It is recommended that the website developer, if using WordPress, use a Yoast or similar SEO plug-in to customize the important SEO information for each page.

- Google Webmaster Tools: Google offers this free tool for developers to determine how much traffic is coming from search terms, identify problems on the website that could be affecting user experience or SEO, and offer valuable documentation for website developers. It will also identify keyword traffic for the website. We recommend that a website developer register each website with the Google Webmaster Toolkit.

BLOGGING FOR SEARCH ENGINE OPTIMIZATION

Blogging, although not mandatory, has become an important component of a modern website. A well-designed blog can help boost the SEO for a website.

One can also keep their website up to date with a blog. A blog is a useful tool to connect with patients by sharing important updates about the practice that do not fall into the category of a procedure page or an about us page. They can also help patients connect with the personal side of the practice or its providers. A blog post could cover the announcement of the launch of a new procedure, an article with advice to patients, or a short story about a personal connection to one of the providers.

A good blog post should contain information that readers want to know. It should not be purely self-promotional information. There is not a fixed rule on length or word count for a blog post. An article can be short with just a few paragraphs or up to several hundred words.

Ideally, it is best to write a new blog article once per month. If one has valuable information to share, he or she can blog up to twice per month for a medical practice. More important than posting multiple times per month is staying on top of the blogging and continuing the blog in the long run. If there are a set of articles that were published close together chronologically but are several years old with no recent activity, this will not give patients a good impression and could negatively affect ratings on Google.

Depending on how well it works with the website design, it can often be beneficial to patients to create a special page on the website that lets visitors see an overview of the blog articles with a little bit of text from the article and links to view each blog post separately. Blogging platforms such as WordPress allow website developers to create categories for the blogs and keyword "tags" for blog posts so that patients can navigate them by the blog topics. Topics can focus around categories of the most important procedures, important information about specific procedures, or provider names. As the number of blog articles grows, a blog can also let patients browse by date ranges.

Blog Posts and Social Media

Some blog posts are naturally linked with social media. In fact, linking back to a blog from certain types of social media posts helps to boost traffic to the website and allows readers of the website to learn more about a topic they discovered on social media. Some social media posts, such as sharing a picture of the staff celebrating a holiday, a reminder of an upcoming event, or other smaller announcements, do not need to be linked back to a blog post.

Common Blogging Pitfalls to Avoid

Although having a blog is beneficial, it can hurt the usability of a website and hurt SEO rankings on Google if done incorrectly. If one repeats content across different blog articles or repeats content verbatim from procedure pages, this will make the website more confusing to navigate and will hurt SEO. If the blog articles contain information that is too unrelated to the website or is off topic, this can hurt SEO as well. More off-topic subjects are best left to social media posts or appended to email blasts if they need to be shared with new patients or the existing patient base. To maintain a high-quality blog, make sure that each article is unique, relevant, and interesting for patients. Examples of blog topics include the following:

- An interview with the doctor about his or her professional training and personal background
- Advice that a provider gives to patients regarding common sources of eye strain and how to avoid these mistakes
- An article regarding the natural process of aging in the eyes and links to procedures that can help

ONLINE CONSULTATIONS

Eye care providers can achieve their marketing goals of a higher conversion rate with effective online communications that have been integrated into the website design. The most important step in providing an effective online consultation is establishing the initial communication. Creating a call to action on the website is a necessary first step for the process. Having a prominent contact form and establishing a secure line of communication are critical.

For eye care, there are many limits to what can be provided in the online consultation, and these limitations should be clearly communicated to the patients. Patients should be able to securely provide their medical information in a HIPAA-compliant online form. Numerous website software tools are available to allow for uploading relevant information digitally in a HIPAA-compliant manner.

After communication with the patient, an online consultation can include providing the patient with recommendations based on the information available, but the goal should be setting up a time for the patient to come into the office. An online consultation may include a video chat with the patient, but research literature on the effectiveness of care provided over video consultation is still sparse.[26]

If the communications take place via email, it is important that the practice email system supports security encryption methods. It is also necessary that the patient initiates the communications and understands the risks of using email as a form of communication for the purpose of handling medical information.

The following guidelines have been assembled for ensuring effective online consultations through the website:

- Establish a secure system for handling communications.
- Offer a personalized response to online inquiries.

- Establish an office process to ensure that each online lead receives a response and that they are tracked for follow-up over time.

- If there are back-and-forth communications with the patient, clarify that to make the best medical recommendations an in-person visit is the next step.

- Because there are limitations to telemedicine in eye care, incorporate the online consultation into a secure lead management system and process at the office to help online contact requests eventually become new patients.

- Allowing patients to leave reviews of their experience with the provider can assist patients in selecting a provider of choice and improve patient experience.[27]

Website visitors can also be invited to join an email marketing list. These lists can be configured to use mail automation to configure a set of messages to periodically touch base or provide important information to the potential new patient.

For an online consultation to be effective, it is important to set the expectation for response time before the patient initializing communications. The office hours should be clearly stated. When patients initiate a request for an online consultation, the form should be open ended to allow patients to clearly communicate their specific concerns.

Another method for patients to consult online with the practice during business hours is a website-embedded online chat tool. This allows patients to receive immediate personalized responses to their questions. Faster responses help maintain or increase patients' satisfaction.

Emerging technologies for initial online communication with patients should be regularly monitored and evaluated. Being responsive to new or different ways that patients prefer to communicate with practices will help eye care providers with their long-term strategy.

REFERENCES

1. Garett R, Chiu J, Zhang L, Young SD. A literature review: website design and user engagement. *Online J Commun Media Technol.* 2016;6(3):1-14.
2. Fogg BJ, Soohoo C, Danielson DR, Marable L, Stanford J, Tauber ER. How do users evaluate the credibility of web sites?: a study with over 2,500 participants. In: *DUX '03: Proceedings of the 2003 Conference on Designing for User Experiences.* ACM; 2013:1-15
3. Martin H. Lawsuits targeting business websites over ADA violations are on the rise. *LA Times.* Published November 11, 2018. Accessed February 27, 2019. https://www.latimes.com/business/la -fi-hotels-ada-compliance-20181111-story.html

4.   Valid HTML statistics. PowerMapper Software. Published January 2018. Accessed February 28, 2019. https://try.powermapper.com/stats/ValidHtmlPages

5.   An D. Find out how you stack up to new industry benchmarks for mobile page speed. Google. Published February 2018. Accessed February 28, 2019. https://www.thinkwithgoogle.com /marketing-resources/data-measurement/mobile-page-speed-new-industry-benchmarks/

6.   Percentage of all global web pages served to mobile phones from 2009 to 2018. Statistica. Published January 2019. Accessed February 28, 2019. https://www.statista.com/statistics/241462/global -mobile-phone-website-traffic-share/

7.   Synder K, Pashmeena H. The changing face of B2B marketing. Google. Published March 2015. Accessed February 28, 2019. https://www.thinkwithgoogle.com/consumer-insights/the-changing -face-b2b-marketing/

8.   Nielsen J. Horizontal attention leans left (early research). Nielsen Normal Group. Published April 6, 2010. Accessed February 20, 2019. https://www.nngroup.com/articles/horizontal-attention -original-research/

9.   Abou-Zahra S, Arch A, Green J, et al. Accessibility: web design and applications. World Wide Web Consortium (W3C). Accessed August 25, 2020. https://www.w3.org/standards/webdesign/ accessibility

10. ADA best practices tool kit for state and local governments. United States Department of Justice Civil Rights Division. Published May 7, 2007. Accessed August 4, 2020. https://www.ada.gov/pca- toolkit/chap5toolkit.htm

11. Abou-Zahra S. Accessibility principles. World Wide Web Consortium (W3C). Updated January 9, 2019. Accessed February 28, 2019. https://www.w3.org/WAI/fundamentals/accessibility-principles/

12. Henry SL. Web content accessibility guidelines (WCAG) overview. World Wide Web Consortium (W3C). Published July 2005. Updated June 22, 2018. Accessed February 20, 2019. https://www.w3 .org/WAI/standards-guidelines/wcag/

13. Report: Gen Z: a look inside its mobile-first mindset. Google. Accessed February 28, 2019. https:// www.thinkwithgoogle.com/interactive-report/gen-z-a-look-inside-its-mobile-first-mindset/

14. Gevelber L. No regrets: the 3 things driving the research-obsessed consumer. Google. Published May 2018. Accessed February 26, 2019. https://www.thinkwithgoogle.com/consumer-insights /consumer-search-behavior/

15. An D, Meenan P. Why marketers should care about mobile page speed. Google. Published July 2016. Accessed February 10, 2019. https://www.thinkwithgoogle.com/marketing-resources /experience-design/mobile-page-speed-load-time/

16. Market share trends for content management systems for websites. W3Techs Web Technology Surveys. Published February 1, 2019. Accessed February 5, 2019. https://w3techs.com/technologies /history_overview/content_management

17. An D. Find out how you stack up to new industry benchmarks for mobile page speed. Google. Published February 2018. Accessed February 28, 2019. https://www.thinkwithgoogle.com /marketing-resources/data-measurement/mobile-page-speed-new-industry-benchmarks/

18. Graham L. The number of devastating cyberattacks is surging—and it's likely to get much worse. CNBC. Published September 20, 2017. Accessed February 22, 2019. https://www.cnbc.com/2017 /09/20/cyberattacks-are-surging-and-more-data-records-are-stolen.html

19. Usage of traffic analysis tools for websites. W3Techs Web Technology Surveys. Updated August 4, 2020. Accessed August 4, 2020. https://w3techs.com/technologies/overview/traffic_analysis/all

20. Kusinitz S. How to decrease your website's bounce rate [infographic]. HubSpot. Published July 17, 2014. Updated May 29, 2018. Accessed August 4, 2020. https://blog.hubspot.com/marketing/ decrease-website-bounce-rate-infographic

21. How Google search works. Google. Accessed February 1, 2019. https://support.google.com /webmasters/answer/70897

22. Shelton K. The value of search results rankings. Forbes. Published October 30, 2017. Accessed February 27, 2019. https://www.forbes.com/sites/forbesagencycouncil/2017/10/30/the-value-of -search-results-rankings/

23. Markup Validation Service. World Wide Web Consortium (W3C). Accessed February 23, 2019. https://validator.w3.org/docs/help.html

24. Jenkinson L, Critchlow T, Chritchlow W, et al. The beginners guide to SEO: chapter 9: myths and misconceptions about search engines. Moz. Accessed August 25, 2020. https://web.archive.org/web/20181116072245/https:/moz.com/beginners-guide-to-seo/myths-and-misconceptions-about-search-engines

25. Toonen E. Does site speed influence SEO? Yoast. Published July 17, 2019. Accessed February 27, 2019. https://yoast.com/does-site-speed-influence-seo/

26. Greenhalgh T, Vijayaraghavan S, Wherton J, et al. Virtual online consultations: advantages and limitations (VOCAL) study. *BMJ Open*. 2016;6:e009388. doi:10.1136/bmjopen-2015-009388

27. Li J, Zhang Y, Ma L, Liu X. The impact of the Internet on health consultation market concentration: an econometric analysis of secondary data. *J Med Internet Res*. 2016;18(10):e276. doi:10.2196/jmir.6423

Vision Seminars as Educational Tools

John Mickner, BA

We have all received emails, texts, or postcards announcing seminars for a product or service. Seminars are a great way for potential patients to learn more about your practice and services offered in an informal setting, usually with refreshments provided. Whether or not you have conducted seminars, the purpose of this chapter is not to give you the best kept secrets of conducting seminars. Rather, it is to illustrate how they can be part of an overall successful marketing strategy and plan. If they are conducted professionally and focused on educating consumers rather than on sales, the result should be prospects for eye care evaluations and eventually contracts for service. On the other hand, if they are unrehearsed, slipshod, and poorly marketed, results will be mediocre and a waste of time, energy, and money. They will get poor results and, even worse, get poor reviews and comments. Over the years, I have either conducted or have been a part of many seminars with varied results. I remember the jubilation when it was standing room only and the frustration when only a few people showed up. In the latter scenario, the atmosphere in the room was

Wang M, ed. *Grow Your Eye Care Practice:*
High-Impact Pearls From the Marketing Experts (pp 105-111).
© 2021 Taylor & Francis Group.

uncomfortable for both my team and the few attendees. The packed room gave the appearance that our firm was successful and must have something worthwhile to offer. The opposite was true with the poorly attended seminar. The appearance was that our firm was not so successful, and attendees may have felt intimidated.

Both types of seminars illustrated were held in the same nice and comfortable meeting room of the same or comparably nice hotels, but the results were drastically different. In both instances, the results had nothing to do with the weather (although sometimes in Pennsylvania it did), time of year, time of day, or day of the week. Poor planning resulted in poor results. Proper planning resulted in much better and often great results. In this chapter, rather than dwelling on the don'ts of vision seminars or any seminar for that matter, I focus on examples of what does work. You can figure out the don'ts yourself based on the examples. For these purposes, the successful examples are based on vision seminars conducted by the Wang Vision Cataract & LASIK Center—An Aier-USA Eye Clinic in Nashville, Tennessee. Dr. Ming Wang and his staff members perform at least 4 different types of LASIK surgeries as well as a full menu of other services to support those patients who do not qualify for LASIK. Whether you are a LASIK surgeon, an optometrist, or an ophthalmologist, if you want to begin offering educational seminars or want to improve on the results of seminars you already offer, this chapter illustrates why Dr. Wang's vision seminars are so successful. I will do my best to not spill any of the "secret sauce" that Dr. Wang and his staff have worked so hard to develop. In fact, if you ever attend one of the Wang Vision Cataract & LASIK Center seminars, the techniques used are self-evident and appreciated by the staff and guests.

Let's talk about that last statement for a second. Why are the marketing techniques used by Wang Vision Cataract & LASIK Center appreciated by the staff and the guests? The following are several reasons that will also help to lead into the actual techniques. The term *guest* is very intentional and will be explained in a minute.

- The staff knows that a successful seminar will increase the potential for scheduling of follow-up eye evaluations, additional LASIK surgeries, and job stability.
- The guests appreciate learning about the various LASIK procedures, hearing testimonies of patients, and getting an explanation of the procedures in order to decide if LASIK surgery is right for them and if it fits into their budget. If everything is explained properly, the results will be scheduled eye evaluations and possibly scheduled surgeries.

In order to get to the end goal of scheduled evaluations and surgeries, a strategy had to be developed and implemented to ensure a successful seminar. First, let's be transparent and honest and recognize the seminars for what they are, namely a sales presentation with the end goals of scheduled eye evaluations, LASIK surgeries, and heartfelt testimonies and referrals by satisfied patients. In order to be successful, the seminars must be a combination of relevant education, fact filled (just enough), and entertaining. Guests do not want to be bombarded with information, especially highly technical and hard-to-understand information. They also do not want to be intimidated or pressured. They do want to be entertained and receive enough valuable information to make a decision. Remember, they are giving up several hours of their evening, and your efforts will be futile if they are not entertained enough to stay for the entire seminar. Let's go through the strategy and implementation of what makes a successful seminar (ie, one that ends with scheduled evaluations on the spot). Remember, people buy products and services based on emotion, and the best time to get guests to schedule evaluations is before they leave the seminar venue.

The successful vision seminar begins with a very deliberate strategy and marketing campaign as follows:

- The meeting location is in a nice hotel with an attractive meeting room capable of seating between 50 and 100 people. The hotel allows food to be brought in; however, Dr. Wang chooses to let the hotel provide the food. Once the food is laid out, the hotel staff only needs to check occasionally to be sure adequate food and beverages are available. When done properly, even pizza and fruit can look elegant.
- The meeting room has excellent, adjustable lighting and is equipped with up-to-date audiovisual equipment, including a large screen and good sound equipment. As a backup, Dr. Wang's staff brings their own microphone and speaker system.
- The meeting room is in an area where the food and registration tables are just outside in a hallway. The registration area is spacious enough to allow guests to sign in at the table and allow others to pass by with ease.
- Seminar signage with Dr. Wang's photo is provided to the hotel and displayed in the lobby near the elevator on a tripod because the seminar is located on an upper floor and, of course, includes the floor number. A smaller copy of the sign is also placed inside the elevator, and a larger sign is placed immediately outside the elevator door on the proper floor with a directional arrow. These details are important. The hotel desk staff is

reminded what floor and room the seminar is being held and what time. There is nothing worse than having a guest ask this information of the hotel staff and be told they have no knowledge of such a seminar.

- The registration table is staffed by vision staff members, so they can answer minor questions by registrants. Staff at the registration table should be cordial and welcoming. They will most likely see these staff members again if they schedule an evaluation.

- The registration table has a tablecloth with the practice/company logo and name, guest registration forms, branded pens and flyers with information about the next upcoming seminar, and Dr. Wang's business cards. The following is an adage that a business consultant friend uses: "It doesn't matter so much who you give your business card to, but rather who they pass it to." The cards and flyers are important.

- The registration form is entitled "Guest Registration Form." If you have been wondering why Dr. Wang addresses attendees as guests, it is for this reason. Part of the success of Disney World/Disneyland is treating park visitors as guests. Guest suggests someone of more importance than just a visitor or attendee. The form has space for the typical things like name, address, phone, and email, but it is also important to ask who invited them to the seminar. Did they find out about the seminar through one or more types of advertising or by referral? If by referral, that person can be thanked for making the referral.

- When guests get their food and enter the meeting room, it is fully lit, and another staff member should greet them and ask how many in their party. This will be important as the room fills and seating gets limited.

- By offering and suggesting preregistration from a link on an email invitation and on the vision center's website, the vision staff knows approximately how many guests to expect. That number of chairs is set up theater style, with a good number stacked up in the back for reserve. It gives the appearance of all chairs being filled and having to add extra.

- There are tall tables in the back of the room for guests to deposit their used dishes and drink glasses/cups.

- The scheduled start time of the seminar is 6:20 to 6:30 PM, allowing 20 to 30 minutes for eating and getting seated, and there is background music playing. Complete silence can be uncomfortable for some. Although guests are waiting for the real show to begin, slides of patients, vision staff, the company offices, and other personally selected photos and short video clips are scrolling in a slideshow. This keeps the guests occupied, and the

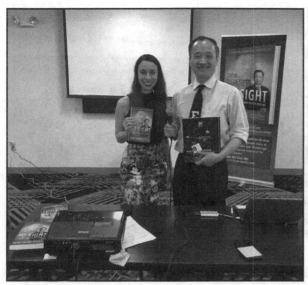

Figure 12-1. Presentations should be set up professionally well before the seminar begins to ensure no issues arise during the seminar.

carefully selected content also demonstrates the friendly atmosphere of the vision center. This preseminar show is also used to specifically show the warm and human side of the doctor who will be performing the surgeries. It is important that staff take care of all the little details like registration, food distribution, guest seating, and audiovisual setup and testing in order to allow Dr. Wang and the emcee to greet and chat with guests for a short time during the preseminar warm-up show (Figure 12-1).

- As the start time gets near, the emcee gives a 10-, 5-, and 2-minute countdown, so guests can make that last restroom visit or get another beverage.
- It is time to start. The emcee, who was chosen for being energetic and enthusiastic, welcomes everyone and mentions that the guests are about to experience the most informative explanation of LASIK and cataract procedures they will ever have and that there will be a drawing at the end of the seminar where several lucky winners will receive a certificate toward discounts on services. It is made crystal clear so that guests understand that to be eligible to win, they must stay until the end, and for those who schedule an evaluation before they leave that evening, the evaluation will be done free of charge. One point of clarification here is needed. The seminar content is indeed most informative and not technically overwhelming.

The seminar includes slides; video clips; and, of course, the verbal comments of the presenter, Dr. Ming Wang. The emcee begins the presentation with a short but complementary bio of the presenter and builds him up to the audience.

Figure 12-2. The room is large enough to fit the expected amount of guests, typically with theater seating.

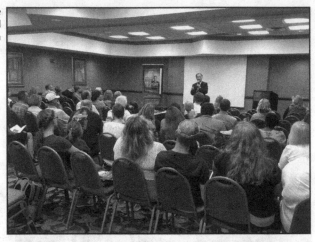

The presenter's job is to display his professionalism and attention to detail by following a precise and well-rehearsed script so that he does not have to think about what he is saying. Everything flows naturally and comes across as a conversation with his guests rather than a sales presentation. This also allows him to be comfortable and to be able to focus on guest reactions and body language. No one would want to go to a Broadway play where each performance was ad-libbed. Remember you are providing a performance, and your performance should be scripted and entertaining, not disjointed and disorganized. The way you present and conduct the seminar, starting way back at registration, will be interpreted as the way you run your practice. When guests leave the seminar well fed; well entertained; and treated professionally, cordially, and respectfully, the odds are greatly increased that they will become patients. It makes them feel important.

As part of the opening comments, Dr. Wang asks several patients to give their brief testimonies to the guests so that they see that others have done what they are considering doing. Dr. Wang asks them specific questions to help them give their testimony because some patients are shy and may have difficulty getting started. These testimonial patients are asked well in advance of the seminar if they would be willing to speak briefly about their experience, and, of course, this guarantees that there will be someone in the room to give a testimony. Dr. Wang then speaks about procedures, medical conditions, and treatments as well as his personal endeavors (Figure 12-2).

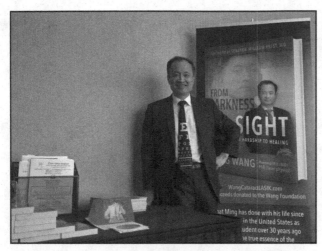

Figure 12-3. Gifts for attendees encourage guests to stay until the end and lend excitement.

As mentioned previously, when the seminar is concluded, the drawing is held to award discount coupons for several lucky guests. This is done formally with some grandiose flair (Figure 12-3). Now that the seminar has been successfully concluded, a reminder about the next seminar is announced while holding up the next seminar flyer. "Please invite family, friends, and coworkers to our next seminar." The guests have just been prompted to be "brand ambassadors" for Wang Vision.

Now the work begins by the staff member or members assigned to seminar marketing for the next seminar. In the interest of keeping this chapter relatively short, suffice it to say that a review of information provided in other chapters related to traditional marketing, search engine optimization, and social media will provide the suggested steps and techniques that can be used to advertise and market the first and subsequent vision seminars.

13

Seasonal Marketing

Michael Malley, BA

CATARACTS

A quick look at your monthly surgical volume for cataract and refractive procedures will affirm there is indeed a seasonality to ophthalmic marketing. Cataract surgical volume starts to trend upward in the fall of each year, peaking somewhere between November and December depending on your holiday and vacation schedule. This phenomenon has less to do with the actual marketing of your cataract practice and more to do with seasonality and, of course, deductibles. That being said, the more you know about the "seasons" of ophthalmic marketing, the more relevant your marketing.

A case in point is the following: Patients previously diagnosed with cataracts who have met their annual deductible by the fall season can save the cost of a new deductible by having their procedure this year. This makes the fall season the most affordable time to have cataract surgery. A sample marketing message

Wang M, ed. *Grow Your Eye Care Practice:*
High-Impact Pearls From the Marketing Experts (pp 113-117).
© 2021 Taylor & Francis Group.

could be as follows: "If you've been diagnosed with a cataract and have met your annual deductible, right now is the most affordable time to have your cataracts removed. A new year means a new deductible." This is a simple and effective message that is straight to the point. This type of seasonal marketing is more educational and informative than traditional offer-based advertising. If done properly, it can be interpreted by the public as a public service to "not wait until the end of the year to schedule their cataract procedure." Typically, by November, surgery schedules begin to fill up, and most surgeons want to take off a week or 2 during the November and December holidays to spend time with their families.

Our firm considers May to be the unofficial start of the cataract marketing season. By that time, most of the seniors who travel south for the winter have returned home. The weather turns favorable for enjoying outdoor activities and favorite hobbies, all of which require good vision. Marketing that reminds people of their need for restored vision to enjoy the things they love most in life actually elevates the perceived value of cataract surgery.

By May, many patients have already met their annual deductibles, making the cost of products like premium lens implants and femtosecond lasers a little more affordable. In an age and time when out-of-pocket expenses for bilateral cataract surgery can range between $2000 and $10,000, perception is reality. If your asking price for cataract surgery does not meet or surpass patients' perceived value, conversion will suffer.

May also represents the ideal season to lead into the American Academy of Ophthalmology's National Cataract Awareness Month in June. Marketing educational awareness allows practices to position themselves as leaders in cataract information and education. Unfortunately, most practices let the month slip by in quiet marketing solitude because they just do not understand the core purpose and benefit of marketing cataract surgery—helping patients make a more informed decision about restoring their vision.

When patients hear that an ophthalmology practice is working in conjunction with an organization like the American Academy of Ophthalmology to help prevent vision loss from cataracts through early diagnosis and treatment, patients interpret that as cataract leadership. They see a practice that is passionate about helping them preserve their vision, a practice that engages in cataract education and is dedicated to community service, and a practice they might even consider when it is time for their cataract procedure. The message starts with basic education and shapes the patients' perspective of the brand.

The most opportune marketing months of the year are a combination of May/June and September/October. In May and June, focus on education and prevention. In September and October, focus on the opportunity to schedule cataract surgery before another annual deductible is required.

Lack of Cataract Marketing

A lack of cataract marketing often results from thinking like a surgeon instead of thinking like a patient. Surgeons think less about informing the general public about the plethora of constantly evolving advancements in cataract surgery and more about the surgical removal of the cataract.

Successful medical marketing occurs when a practice gives the public information it wants to hear, not a message a surgeon or practice wants to say. A surgeon may want to talk about methods of cataract extraction or implantation. A patient may want to hear why early diagnosis and treatment are important. A surgeon may want to discuss the variations in lens implant design. A patient may want to hear how cataracts are formed and if everyone eventually develops them.

Basic cataract education will always be well received by the general public. Recent advancements in cataract care will always be welcomed by cataract patients as well. It simply must be delivered on their level in a format they easily understand. Few practices outside of the Florida market even engage in cataract marketing regardless of the seasonal opportunities. They simply wait for patients to be referred to their practice or hope patients find them online.

LASIK/REFRACTIVE

The season for LASIK is not quite as defined or limited as cataract marketing. In some cases, the timing can almost be the opposite. For instance, January and February have traditionally been 2 of the highest LASIK volume surgical months. This spike in volume could be traced to men and women wanting to use their flex spending account (FSA) or their health savings account (HSA) funds as early into the new year as possible.

Others considering LASIK in January and February were doing so because they simply wanted to begin their new year by kicking off their glasses and contacts for LASIK. Marketing messaging for LASIK in January and February could be "Enjoy new vision in the New Year by using your Flex Spending Account or your Health Savings Account dollars for 'Tax-Free' LASIK." Because the FSA and HSA tax benefits have been reduced, the percentage of patients timing their LASIK procedures in January and February to take full advantage of those benefits early has declined. However, promoting these tax-free LASIK benefits is still a viable strategy at seasonal times of the year.

In addition to reminding potential LASIK patients of how easy it is to keep a New Year's resolution of freedom from glasses or contacts in the new year and the tax-free benefits, a second seasonal opportunity for FSA and HSA messaging is the fall. It is important to remind patients they will lose their FSA benefit if they do not use it on a procedure like LASIK. Each fall consider running a "use it or lose it" campaign for LASIK. This message can also be effective during the holiday season in November and December. Include a reminder that FSA dollars can also be used for contacts, glasses (including computer glasses), and sun wear.

Although seasonal LASIK marketing is not tied to deductibles and insurance coverages like cataract surgery, it can also be effective with unique creative messaging and specific offers developed for each season. Spring is a time for renewal, so remind potential patients of the "need to renew their vision with LASIK." Summertime is no time for glasses and contacts, so turn "summer time" into "LASIK time." Fall is all about change and "What better way to change your life than with LASIK?" Never let your marketing team forget that the ultimate gift every holiday season is the gift of sight.

PEDIATRICS AND SCHOOL EXAMS

The 6 weeks before the start of school is an extremely busy time for students to renew their glasses and contact prescriptions. College students, in particular, often schedule visits before leaving for fall semester classes as well as over winter break. Marketing messages about vision and education, sports and eyewear, and back to school exams work well during June and July.

DESIGNATED VISION MONTHS

Certain months have been chosen as celebratory months for eye care. January is Glaucoma Awareness Month. February is Age-Related Macular Degeneration Awareness Month. March is Workplace Eye Wellness Month. April is Sports Eye Safety Month. May is Healthy Vision Month. June is Fireworks Eye Safety and Cataract Awareness Month. July is Ultraviolet Safety Month. August is Children's Eye Health and Safety Month, as well as Dry Eye Awareness Month. September is Healthy Aging Month. October is Halloween Safety Month. November is Diabetic Eye Disease Awareness Month, and December is Safe Toys and Celebrations Month. Educational messages on these timely topics work well in marketing messages.

Seasonal cataract and refractive marketing can be a fun, rewarding, topical, and timely way to market your services in a manner that patients will appreciate. Seasonal marketing allows your messaging to remain fresh. Most people enjoy the beginning of a new season but lose their seasonal enthusiasm toward the end. This is especially true in the later parts of winter and the longer, hotter parts of summer. Make sure your seasonal messaging is designed around the front end of each season.

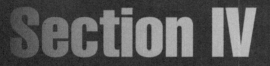

Section IV

The Laws and Ethics That Regulate Health Care Marketing

14

Marketing Laws

James E. Looper Jr, JD; Tracy Schroeder Swartz, OD, MS, FAAO, Dipl ABO;
and Ming Wang, MD, PhD

Many industries other than health care enjoy wide latitude in how they can legally advertise. In contrast, many common marketing practices that are legal in other industries are strictly prohibited within the health care industry. Under federal and state law, claims in health care marketing materials generally must be truthful and evidence based and cannot be deceptive or unfair. When advertising as a physician, it is vitally important to comply with truth-in-advertising standards. In addition to supporting advertising claims with evidence, physician marketing must follow the rules and regulations specific to health care or face serious consequences.

GENERAL MARKETING LAWS

According to the American Marketing Association, "Marketing communications, or 'marcom,' is an all-encompassing term, as it covers marketing

Wang M, ed. *Grow Your Eye Care Practice:*
High-Impact Pearls From the Marketing Experts (pp 121-132).
© 2021 Taylor & Francis Group.

practices and tactics including advertising, branding, graphic design, promotion, publicity, public relations and more."[1] As evident by the breadth of this definition, there is great potential to run afoul of marketing law pitfalls even if one is not intentionally engaging in marketing activities. Therefore, a basic understanding of marketing law is necessary to avoid potential civil or criminal penalties.

Marketing is simply the act of relaying information about a product or service to the general public by the provider of the service or product, and for many business owners, even those within the medical field, it is the key to success. However, every business has a legal obligation to ensure that its marketing materials are truthful and not in violation of the law. Marketing law refers generally to a body of law composed of the statutes, rules and regulations, and associated case law concerned with preventing consumer harm from deceptive marketing practices in the sale of goods and services.[2] As a result, it tends to be particularly strict with regard to medical services, drugs, and medical devices.

In the United States, the Federal Trade Commission (FTC) is the federal agency responsible for regulating advertisers. The FTC is responsible for enforcing the marketing law in place today along with creating new rules and regulations.

Truth in advertising refers to the body of law governing truthful marketing. These laws cover the following communications:

- Health claims: These are rules and regulations concerning the reported effects for products such as glaucoma drugs, antiaging products, and supplements. Similarly, this section would cover disclosing results from surgical procedures.

- Product endorsements: These include rules and regulations requiring that a celebrity's endorsements be truthful if the celebrity decides to endorse a product. The endorsement must reflect the honest opinions, findings, beliefs, and/or experience of the endorser. The celebrity must have actually used the product while the advertisement is running.[3]

- Advertising to children: These are rules designed to prevent communicating misleading information to impressionable young people.

- "Made in the USA" labels: These are rules and regulations stating how much or what percentage of a product must be created in the United States before a company can label its product in this manner.

- Environmental impact: This includes rules and regulations related to environmental impact claims or benefit of a product. For example, information regarding the content of recycled material in a product labeled "recycled" would fall under this category.

MEDICARE AND MEDICAID ANTI-KICKBACK STATUTE

The Anti-Kickback Statute (AKS) is an intent-based statute that contains both civil and criminal penalties and, depending on how the activity is undertaken, may also affect some marketing activities. The AKS is not limited to marketing activities that may be implicated by any arrangement in which anything of value changes hands between a referral source and a third party in relation to the provision of services paid for by a federal program. However, some practices that otherwise may run afoul of the statute are protected. Certain regulations were developed to protect various payment and business practices. These protected practices are known as *safe harbor regulations*. Under a safe harbor regulation, the protected practice is not treated as a criminal offense under the law. On the other hand, if an arrangement falls outside the safe harbor, although it may not be illegal, the circumstances behind the arrangement should be carefully reviewed. Marketing may include activities to increase business through incentives, which may implicate the AKS.

A common situation in which many physicians find themselves in is when they entertain and present gifts to potential referral sources. Physicians and other health care providers must be aware that these types of activities fall squarely within the ambit of the AKS.[4] To help avoid violations, the Office of the Inspector General has issued compliance guidance that addresses entertainment and gifts. The Office of the Inspector General has suggested that gifts, gratuities, and other entertainment activities significantly raise the risk of violating the AKS when these activities involve individuals who may be positioned to refer services or to influence potential referrals to a health care provider.

Physicians should never provide cash gifts to referral sources. Additionally, nonmonetary gifts cannot be tied or attached to referrals, must be of nominal value (extremely low or almost no real value), and should be associated with educational or business activities and sessions. Should a physician take a referral source to dinner, a significant portion of time should be spent discussing business and/or education topics. The physician should be mindful of the amount spent at said dinner as well as the amount spent over the course of the year on this referral source.

If a physician hires a marketing representative, a physician liaison, or a similar employee or used a contracted employee to provide marketing services for the practice, compensation cannot be connected to the number of referrals made. Aggregate compensation paid to the employee or contractor should be set in advance, and it should be consistent with fair market value. If the physician employs rather than independently contracts with the marketing representative, the AKS provides more flexibility. The safe harbor related to employees allows the employer to pay an employee any amount for his or her employment services, which permits percentage-based compensation. The physician can only take advantage of the safe harbor if the employee is truly an employee as defined and determined by the Internal Revenue Service.

Many recent settlements concerning the AKS involve staggering numbers. For illustration, a subsidiary of Community Health Systems, Health Management Associates, agreed to pay the federal government $262 million to settle fraudulent billing and kickback allegations. Health Management Associates was alleged to have billed government payers incorrectly for inpatient services that should have been billed as less costly observation or outpatient services, paid physicians in exchange for referrals, and submitted claims to Medicare and Medicaid for falsely inflated emergency department facility fee charges.[5]

On a smaller scale, another settlement amounted to $20.7 million for violation of the AKS and Stark Law (covered later). This lawsuit was originally brought under the whistleblower provisions of the False Claims Act by Tullio Emanuele, MD, in 2010. Dr. Emanuele worked for Medicor from 2001 to 2005. In the lawsuit, he alleged the Hamot Medical Center paid Medicor up to $2 million per year from 1999 to 2010 under services arrangements to secure patient referrals from Medicor.[6]

STARK LAW

The Stark Law prohibits physicians from making referrals for certain designated health services payable by Medicare to an entity to which they or a family member has a financial relationship. Designated health services examples that apply to this law include inpatient and outpatient services, laboratory services, physical therapy, radiology, and home health services. Intent is not required for penalty.[7]

Under this law, there is an exception for nonmonetary compensation that applies to certain marketing activities commonly used by physicians. Under the exception, physicians who furnish meals or noncash gifts such as event tickets to a referring physician up to an annual limit of approximately $423 (in 2020, adjusted for inflation annually) will be protected.[8] In addition, the following criteria must be met:

- The compensation is not determined by the volume or value of referrals or other business generated by the referring physician.
- The compensation may not be solicited by the physician or the physician's practice, including employees and staff members.
- The compensation arrangement does not violate the AKS or any federal or state law or regulation governing billing or claims submission.[7]

The dollar limit for "medical staff incidental benefits" such as meals, parking, and other incidental items or services used is less than $36 per occurrence for 2020.[8] If a physician's marketing activities do not comply with this exception and more money is given to the referral source, the paying physician will not be able to lawfully bill for any designated health services ordered by that referring physician or source.

If a physician inadvertently provides nonmonetary compensation to a referring physician in excess of the annual limit, such compensation is deemed to be within the $423 limit if (1) the value of the excess nonmonetary compensation is no more than 50% of the annual limit, and (2) the referring physician returns the excess nonmonetary compensation (or an amount equal to the value of the excess nonmonetary compensation) to the paying physician.[8]

The return must be made by the end of the calendar year in which the excess nonmonetary compensation was received or within 180 consecutive calendar days after the date the excess nonmonetary compensation was received by the physician, whichever is earlier. This return option may be used by an entity only once every 3 years with respect to the same referring physician.[7]

Penalties include civil monetary fines of up to $15,000 per service as well as higher penalties for circumvention schemes. In addition, physicians and other entities that are in contravention of the law can forfeit their right to participate in Medicare and Medicaid provider programs.

We discuss in depth the payment of comanagement fees here. An example of a violation of Stark Law resulting in a penalty can be found in a settlement with Aurora Health Care (Milwaukee, Wisconsin). Aurora Health Care agreed to pay $12 million to settle allegations it violated the False Claims Act and Stark Law.[9] Aurora allegedly entered into compensation arrangements with 2 physicians that violated Stark Law because the arrangements were not commercially reasonable and because they took into account the physicians' anticipated referrals. According to the Justice Department, the compensation also exceeded the fair market value of the physicians' services and was not for identifiable services. Aurora submitted claims for services ordered by the 2 physicians to Medicare and Medicaid, which is illegal.

In another recent example, in June 2018, federal prosecutors unsealed charges against 9 defendants for their alleged roles in a kickback scheme resulting in the submission of more than $950 million in fraudulent claims. The defendants were charged after the government's investigation into the kickbacks the physicians received for patient referrals for spinal surgeries performed at Pacific Hospital in Long Beach, California. Daniel Capen, MD, an orthopedic surgeon, agreed to plead guilty to conspiracy and illegal kickback charges. He allegedly submitted about $142 million of Pacific Hospital's claims to insurers. Timothy Hunt, MD, who allegedly referred spinal surgery patients for surgery, agreed to plead guilty to a conspiracy charge involving his receipt of illegal kickbacks. Tiffany Rogers, MD, also allegedly received illegal kickbacks to refer patients for spinal surgeries to Pacific Hospital. The former chief financial officer of Pacific Hospital's physician management department, George Hammer, agreed to plead guilty to tax charges based on the fraudulent classification of illegal kickbacks in hospital-related corporate tax filings. Two chiropractors as well as 2 companies and an individual associated with one of the chiropractors were also charged for their alleged involvement. Michael Drobot, former owner and chief executive officer of Pacific Hospital, orchestrated the 15-year-long kickback scheme and was sentenced to more than 5 years in prison.[10]

HEALTH INSURANCE PORTABILITY AND ACCOUNTABILITY ACT PRIVACY RULE AND MARKETING

The Privacy Rule addresses the use of protected health information for marketing purposes by the following:

- Defining the term *marketing* under the rule
- Excepting from that definition certain treatment or health care operations activities
- Requiring individual authorization for all uses or disclosures of protected health information for marketing purposes with limited exceptions[11]

The Privacy Rule defines marketing as making "a communication about a product or service that encourages recipients of the communication to purchase or use the product or service."[11] If the communication is marketing, then the communication can occur only if the physician first obtains the patient's authorization. For example, a communication is emailed from an ophthalmologist informing former patients about an outpatient surgery facility that is not part of his or her practice that can provide a baseline fundus photo for $25. This communication is not for the purpose of providing treatment advice but rather for marketing the fundus camera.

Under the Privacy Rule, marketing also means:

> An arrangement between a covered entity and any other entity whereby the covered entity discloses protected health information to the other entity, in exchange for direct or indirect remuneration, for the other entity or its affiliate to make a communication about its own product or service that encourages recipients of the communication to purchase or use that product or service.[11]

This part of the definition to marketing has no exceptions. Patients must authorize these marketing communications before they occur. A physician may not sell protected health information to another party for that party's own purposes. In addition, physicians may not sell lists of patients or enrollees to third parties without obtaining authorization from each person on the list. For example, a physician must obtain permission to give a supplement company patients' emails or phone numbers before sending that information to the supplement company.

The Privacy Rule also defines what is considered "not marketing." This includes communications made to describe a health-related product or service or payment for such product or service that is provided by, or included in a plan of benefits of, the physician making the communication. This would include communications about the physician participating in a health care provider network or health plan network; replacement of, or enhancements to, a health plan; and health-related products or services available only to a health plan enrollee that add value to, but are not part of, a plan of benefits. This exception to the marketing definition permits communications by a covered entity about its own products or services.[11]

A communication is not marketing if it is made for treatment of the individual.[11] For example, under this exception, it is not marketing, and authorization is not required when a pharmacy or other health care provider mails prescription refill reminders to patients or if an optometrist refers a patient to a glaucoma specialist for an evaluation or provides free samples of a glaucoma drug to a patient.

The third exception is a communication made for case management or care coordination for the individual or to direct or recommend alternative treatments, therapies, health care providers, or settings of care to the individual.[11]

For example, under this exception, an optometrist shares a patient's medical record with several refractive surgeons to determine which technology is best for the patient's case.

For any of these 3 exceptions to the definition of marketing, the activity must otherwise be permissible under the Privacy Rule, and a covered entity may use a business associate to make the communication.[11] As with any disclosure to a business associate, the covered entity must obtain the business associate's agreement to use the protected health information only for the communication activities of the covered entity before divulging the information.

A communication does not require an authorization, even if it is marketing, if it is in the form of a face-to-face communication by a physician to an individual or a promotional gift of nominal value provided by the physician. For example, giving a cataract patient a vinyl bag with artificial tears, a shield, tape, and sunglasses personally at the time of surgery does not require authorization.

CHILDREN AND THE LAW

The Children's Online Privacy Protection Act was enacted in 1998. If you market to children or use photos of children, this rule would apply. The Children's Online Privacy Protection Act required the FTC to issue and enforce regulations concerning children's online privacy. Although it became effective on April 21, 2000, the FTC issued an amended rule on December 19, 2012, which took effect on July 1, 2013. The rule was designed to protect children under 13 years of age. The rule applies to operators of commercial websites and online services including mobile applications. It applies to services directed to children under 13 years of age that collect, use, or disclose personal information from children. It also applies to operators of general audience websites or online services with actual knowledge that they are collecting, using, or disclosing personal information from children under 13 years of age and websites or online services that have actual knowledge that they are collecting personal information directly from users of another website or online service directed to children. Operators covered by the rule must do the following:

- Post a clear and comprehensive online privacy policy describing their information practices for personal information collected online from children.
- Provide direct notice to parents and obtain verifiable parental consent, with limited exceptions, before collecting personal information online from children.

- Give parents the choice of consenting to the operator's collection and internal use of a child's information but prohibiting the operator from disclosing that information to third parties (unless disclosure is integral to the site or service, in which case, this must be made clear to parents).

- Provide parents access to their child's personal information to review and/or have the information deleted.

- Give parents the opportunity to prevent further use or online collection of a child's personal information.

- Maintain the confidentiality, security, and integrity of information they collect from children, including by taking reasonable steps to release such information only to parties capable of maintaining its confidentiality and security.

- Retain personal information collected online from a child for only as long as is necessary to fulfill the purpose for which it was collected and delete the information using reasonable measures to protect against its unauthorized access or use.[12]

The most likely issue related to this law is a child's photograph. If you have collected photos or videos containing a child's image before the effective date of the amended rule, you do not need to obtain parental consent. However, as a best practice, the FTC recommends that entities either discontinue the use or disclosure of such information after the effective date of the amended rule or, if possible, obtain parental consent.

FEDERAL TRADE COMMISSION REGULATIONS SPECIFIC TO REFRACTIVE EYE SURGERY

In 2008, the FTC prepared guidance on marketing LASIK and other refractive procedures. This document specified Section 5 of the FTC Act prohibits deceptive or unfair practices in or affecting commerce, and Section 12 prohibits the dissemination of any false advertisement to induce the purchase of any food, drug, device, or service.[13] An advertisement is deceptive under Section 5 of the FTC Act if it has a statement, or omits information, that is likely to mislead consumers acting reasonably under the circumstances, and it is important to a consumer's decision to buy or use the product. This act specifies an ad or business practice is unfair if "it causes or is likely to cause substantial consumer injury that a consumer could not reasonably avoid; and the injury is not outweighed by any benefit the practice provides to consumers or competition."[12]

The act also clarified both "express" and "implied" claims that may be made in advertising. An express claim is made literally in the ad. For example, claiming in an advertisement that "more of our World's Best LASIK Center patients achieve 20/20 vision than anyone else" is an express claim. An implied claim is made by inference and is indirect. For example, a patient stating "the procedure was easy, and I saw perfectly immediately afterward" implies a lack of complications and/or side effects for most of World's Best LASIK Center's patients. Physicians must have proof to back up any claim that consumers reasonably take from any marketing material used. Claims that convey an inaccurate impression about refractive surgery's safety, efficacy, success, or other benefits would concern the FTC. For example, claiming wavefront LASIK procedures will allow patients to "throw away their eyeglasses" may be deceptive without further qualification. Furthermore, claims regarding surgical success rates, long-term visual stability, or predictability of surgical outcome must be substantiated by competent and reliable scientific evidence.[13]

The FTC also considers what is not said, and it looks for omitted information that may mislead prospective patients. For example, if an advertisement stated "Call for a free consultation," it must also be stated that a comprehensive examination is required before surgery.

Lawsuits

The risk of health care marketing involves an increased risk in lawsuits. Issues may include copyright infringement, trademarks, and Health Insurance Portability and Accountability Act violations. Lawsuits may be avoided with proper education and compliance training, but consultation with a lawyer is recommended.

Marketers who fail to perform due diligence before using images, articles, or copy that belongs to others put themselves at greater risk for a lawsuit. Even nonwillful infringement may be liable for statutory damages of considerable amounts.

Trademark oppositions are contested proceedings before the US Trademark Trial and Appeal Board. A trademark opposition is typically filed when an applicant did not perform a proper trademark search and clearance before launching his or her brand or marketing campaign. A contested trademark opposition proceeding may cost over $75,000 in attorney's fees.

Trademark infringement actions are adjudicated before the US federal and state courts. If a doctor is found liable for infringement, he or she may be liable for treble (ie, 3 times the amount) damages in exceptional cases as well as the other side's attorney's fees (https://www.healthcaremarketinglaw.com/).[1]

Compliance Programs

As a health care entity pursuing trade marking, it is recommended that a trademark education and compliance program for employees be implemented.[14] Suggestions for areas covered in the compliance program include the following:

- Trademark definitions and concepts
- Explanation of the trademark clearance process
- How to search, clear, and apply to register trademarks
- Trademark use guidelines
- What is and is not trademark fair use
- Employee roles, responsibilities, and procedures
- Creative and marketing vendor responsibilities and procedures
- Trademark usage in digital marketing, including paid search

Risk and compliance training should take place with both employees and vendors responsible for brand assets, marketing, and promotions annually to mitigate risk.

KNOW YOUR STATE LAWS

The state board of medicine may have specific laws of which each licensed physician should be aware. These can be found on each state's medical board website and are also listed at https://www.etnainteractive.com/blog/medical-marketing-laws/. These should be reviewed periodically to ensure one is up to date with the most recent rules and regulations.

REFERENCES

1. Hastings J. Health marcom legal risks in 2019. Collen: Healthcare Marketing Law Guide. Published January 10, 2019. Accessed August 25, 2020. https://www.healthcaremarketinglaw.com/2019/01/health-marcom-legal-trends-in-2019/

2. Marketing law. HG.org Legal Resources. Updated 2020. Accessed August 5, 2020. https://www.hg.org/marketing-law.html

3. Title 16. Chapter I. Subchapter B. Part 255. 38 Stat. 717, as amended; 15 U.S.C. 41 - 58. 74 FR 53138, October 15, 2009. Updated August 3, 2020. Accessed August 5, 2020. https://www.ecfr.gov/cgi-bin/text-idx?SID=701066299822530421fece37367c91d3&mc=true&node=pt16.1.255&rgn=div5

4. Dresvic A. Key regulations impacting healthcare marketing: entertainment and gifts. Published 2010. Accessed August 5, 2020. https://www.thehealthlawpartners.com/files/rbma.january-february_2010.key_regulations_impacting_healthcare_marketing_-_entertainment_and_gifts.pdf

5.   Ellison A. Legal & regulatory issues: CHS subsidiary to pay $262M to settle fraud probe. Published September 26, 2018. Accessed March 2, 2019. https://www.beckershospitalreview.com/legal-regulatory-issues/chs-unit-to-pay-262m-to-settle-fraud-probe.html

6.   Ellison A. Legal & regulatory issues: UPMC Hamot, cardiology practice ink $20.7M settlement in kickback case. Published March 8, 2018. Accessed March 2, 2019. https://www.beckershospitalreview.com/legal-regulatory-issues/upmc-cardiology-practice-ink-20-7m-settlement-in-kickback-case.html

7.   Render H. 2019 Non-monetary compensation to physicians (and chance to review 2018). Health Law News. Published December 19, 2018. Accessed August 5, 2020. https://www.hallrender.com/2018/12/19/2019-non-monetary-compensation-to-physicians-and-chance-to-review-2018/

8.   Centers for Medicare and Medicaid Services. CPI-U updates: non-monetary compensation and medical staff incidental benefits exceptions. Updated Decmeber 20, 2019. Accessed August 25, 2020.

9.   Ellison A. Legal & regulatory issues: Aurora Health will pay $12M to resolve improper compensation claims. Published December 13, 2018. Accessed March 2, 2019. https://www.beckershospitalreview.com/legal-regulatory-issues/aurora-health-will-pay-12m-to-resolve-improper-compensation-claims.html

10. Ellison A. Legal & regulatory issues: ex-CFO, 3 surgeons charged in $950M kickback scheme in California. Published June 29, 2018. Accessed March 2, 2019. https://www.beckershospitalreview.com/legal-regulatory-issues/ex-cfo-3-surgeons-charged-in-950m-kickback-scheme-in-california.html

11. 45 CFR 164.501, 164.508(a)(3).

12. Complying with COPPA: frequently asked questions. Accessed March 2, 2019. https://www.ftc.gov/tips-advice/business-center/guidance/complying-coppa-frequently-asked-questions#General Questions

13. Marketing of refractive eye care surgery: guidance for eye care providers. Accessed March 4, 2019. https://www.ftc.gov/tips-advice/business-center/guidance/marketing-refractive-eye-care-surgery-guidance-eye-care

14. Hastings J. Health system trademark compliance. Collen: Healthcare Marketing Law Guide. Published July 9, 2018. Assessed August 5, 2020. https://www.healthcaremarketinglaw.com/category/hipaa-marketing/

15

Ethics and Marketing

James E. Looper Jr, JD; Tracy Schroeder Swartz, OD, MS, FAAO, Dipl ABO;
and Ming Wang, MD, PhD

Prior to 1982, the American Medical Association's Code of Medical Ethics restricted physicians from advertising. In 1982, the Federal Trade Commission (FTC) won a lawsuit against the American Medical Association, which resulted in physicians being permitted to market health care services. Since that lawsuit, health care marketing has grown by leaps and bounds. Unfortunately, this growth has led to ethical gray areas regarding what should be permitted in health care advertisements and the promotion of products and services.

In previous sections and chapters, we have already discussed some of the applicable marketing laws that govern what you should and may do in regard to marketing. In this chapter, we focus on what not to do by discussing several examples of unethical marketing.

Wang M, ed. *Grow Your Eye Care Practice:*
High-Impact Pearls From the Marketing Experts (pp 133-145).
© 2021 Taylor & Francis Group.

Do Not Exaggerate or Make False Claims

Rule number one is avoid making exaggerated, unverified, and/or false claims. When Tec Laboratories and CleanWell claimed their hand sanitizers could prevent infection from methicillin-resistant *Staphylococcus aureus*, the FTC sent both companies a warning letter requesting that they withdraw these claims from their marketing materials.[1]

In another example, ads for Airborne (Schiff Vitamins) claimed that their supplement was an "herbal health formula that boosts your immune system to help your body combat germs," including germs that caused the common cold. An ABC News investigation from 2006 found that the clinical study Airborne used to prove its cold-fighting abilities was conducted by 2 laypersons hired explicitly to conduct the study, and the study never involved any scientists or doctors. The Center for Science in the Public Interest led a class action suit against Airborne in 2008, which resulted in a $23 million settlement.

When research is referenced in marketing communications, it must substantiate the claims being made. Research data substantiating claims may be requested by the US Food and Drug Administration (FDA) during an investigation. For example, the FDA requested information from Eisai Inc related to its Dacogen product. Dacogen is used to treat blood cell disorders. Salespeople distributed a patient brochure to medical practitioners that claimed 38% of study patients had a positive response to the drug. The FDA found that statistic was taken from a small subgroup of patients who responded well to the drug. When all the patients actually enrolled into the study were included, the response rate was actually 20%. As a result, the FDA sent them a warning letter in November 2009.

Do Not Plagiarize

When creating a website or campaign, do not plagiarize other marketing communications. Website information and marketing material should be original.

Do Not Intentionally Mislead

Do not distort facts or intentionally mislead people. One example is Ferrero's claim that their hazelnut spread Nutella contained "simple, quality ingredients like hazelnuts, skim milk and a hint of cocoa"[2] despite having 21 grams of sugar and 200 calories in each 2-tablespoon serving. The makers of Nutella settled the lawsuit for $3 million. Similarly, in 2010, the FTC announced that Kellogg's claims that Rice Krispies boost a child's immunity with "25 percent Daily Value of Antioxidants and Nutrients—Vitamins A, B, C and E" were "dubious" and ordered the company to discontinue all advertising stating these claims.[3]

Even with limited statements in the advertisement, the pictures in connection with statements must be an accurate depiction and may not be misleading. For example, in 2009, an advertisement for Olay Definity eye cream showed a picture of model Twiggy looking wrinkle free reportedly due to her use of the product. It turned out the ads were retouched.[4] Photoshopping or enhancing photographs is unethical.

In November 2018, FDA issued a warning letter to Electric Lotus, LLC for selling e-liquids (substances used in e-cigarettes) that resemble kid-friendly foods, such as cereal or candy. The e-liquid images were sold in packages that resembled Cinnamon Toast Crunch (General Mills), Lucky Charms (General Mills), and Rice Krispies Treats (Kellogg's) cereals; some of the images resembled LifeSavers candies (Wrigley Company).[5] In response, the offending products were removed from the market.

DO NOT OVERCHARGE

Do not charge significantly more than the actual product or service. Prices of offers must be equal or less than the value to the patient. One example of price inflation was Dannon's Activia yogurt. In 2010, Dannon advertised its probiotic yogurt as "clinically" and "scientifically proven" to boost your immune system and able to help to regulate digestion. Dannon also priced their Activia products at 30% higher prices than other yogurt products. A lawsuit against Dannon was filed in 2008, resulting in a $45 million fine. Dannon was ordered to remove "clinically" and "scientifically proven" from its product labels.[6]

In 2014, Walmart advertised a nationwide sale of Coca-Cola in which 12-packs would cost just $3.00. However, in New York State, customers were charged $3.50 for a 12-pack. Walmart staff allegedly told customers that New York had a "sugar tax" and that the national ad campaign did not apply in New York State. New York Attorney General Eric Schneiderman's investigation into the sales found that the 16% markup above the advertised price violates New York State's General Business Law 349 and 350. Walmart agreed to pay over $66,000 in fines.[7]

DO NOT HIDE POTENTIAL SIDE EFFECTS

Do not conceal potentials side effects or downsides to a treatment or medical service. A pertinent example of this was the FDA's report and subsequent warning letter to Allergan regarding Latisse (bimatoprost). In 2009, the FDA warned Allergan that its website failed to educate consumers regarding the risks of using Latisse, and it used wording that was misleading.[8]

In 2010, the FDA warned Eli Lilly for failing to prominently include risk information in its printed advertisements for Cymbalta. In one advertisement, the drug's treatment prominently featured a woman suffering from chronic knee pain. Information about the drug's risks, including nausea, insomnia, diarrhea, and suicidal ideation, were not listed on the same page. Instead, the risks appeared on an adjacent page.[9]

DO NOT REFLECT NEGATIVELY ON COMPETITORS

Do not bad mouth or gossip about rivals. Instead, educate about your services and why you are the better choice by promoting positive information about yourself.

DO NOT USE SEX SYMBOLS OR PRESSURE SELLING

Do not use sex symbols in marketing for health care. Marketing health care should focus on product or services only. One recent example, albeit not health care but similar, is the lawsuit against Justin Timberlake and Bai Brands. A lawsuit was filed in 2018 by a California man who states the manufacturers of Bai Brands beverages touted their drinks as all natural when they actually contain undisclosed artificial flavors in violation of state and federal law.[10] Not only was Timberlake a spokesperson at the time, he was named "chief flavor officer" in 2016.

Do not use limited-time offers or insist the patient make a decision immediately to secure a product or service.

Do Not Discriminate

If marketing communications convey people of a certain race, age, sex, or religion are superior to others, they are unethical. For example, a PlayStation (Sony Interactive Entertainment) billboard in Europe read "White is coming" next to an image of a white woman viciously holding a shorter black woman. Another example is the Intel advertisement depicting a tall white man surrounded by 6 African American men kneeling at his feet with the following text: "Multiply computing performance and maximize the power of your employees."[11]

Do Not Spam

Do not send unsolicited emails to encourage the use of services or purchase of products.[12] Furthermore, in the health care context, this may be a Health Insurance Portability and Accountability Act (HIPAA) violation if performed without authorization.

Do Not Attempt to Manipulate Search Engines

There are also some unethical activities specific to website management and search engine optimization. Do not duplicate the content on another website. Content should be original to your site. Shadow domains, or domains that drive traffic to your page, are deceptive and should not be used. Keywords or an overabundance of tags will not only make the site look unprofessional but also will not get the attention of modern search engines. Do not hide text in the margins or footers.[13] So-called *black hat* link building actions, such as spamming other sites' comment sections or forum threads or hacking websites to place self-serving links on another site, are unethical.

Another Ethical Issue: Comanagement

Although eye care practitioners may not consider comanagement marketing, the Centers for Medicare & Medicaid Services and others might disagree. In 1992, the Centers for Medicare & Medicaid Services focused on global surgery billing for major surgeries, including ophthalmic procedures. Global periods include preoperative, intraoperative, and postoperative care, which can be billed together or separately. When dividing billing of services for global surgeries, preoperative and intraoperative services are valued at 80% of the total global cost, whereas postoperative services are valued at 20%.[14] In 2000, the Office of the Inspector General (OIG) revised the referral arrangement safe harbor and took a strong stance against the routine agreements between ophthalmologists and optometrists to split global surgery fees. The OIG stated the referral arrangement safe harbor does not protect referral arrangements when physicians bill Medicare using the 54/55 modifiers to indicate an 80/20 split of the global fee for cataract surgery.[15] Although the OIG did not declare such arrangements illegal, it stated these arrangements would be analyzed case by case.

In 2000, the American Society of Cataract and Refractive Surgery (ASCRS) and the American Academy of Ophthalmology (AAO) published a joint paper declaring comanagement should be undertaken only as an exceptional occurrence. Both the AAO and ASCRS advocated for comanagement of postoperative care only when the surgeon was unavailable or the patient was unable to travel to the surgeon's office. The American Optometric Association (AOA) responded by publishing a paper titled "Optometric Postoperative Care," refuting AAO and ASCRS's stance on comanagement.[16] The AOA claimed AAO and ASCRS's position on comanagement was not supported by ethics rules or federal guidance or laws. The AOA suggested ethics and laws be followed to meet the objectives of good patient care.

On October 7, 2011, the OIG issued an opinion permitting a comanagement arrangement involving patients who received conventional and premium intraocular lenses (IOLs). When a Medicare beneficiary elects to receive a premium IOL during cataract surgery, Medicare will pay for the surgery and the amount of the conventional IOL. In this case, the beneficiary is responsible for the difference in cost between the conventional and premium IOL along with the professional and facility fees related to the additional testing and other services related to the correction of refractive errors.[17] This 2011 advisory opinion indicated arrangements in which an optometrist may bill a fee for services not covered by the Medicare program in connection with cataract surgery and comanagement are permitted.

In 2016, the AAO published the Comprehensive Guidelines for Comanagement of Ophthalmic Postoperative Care.[18] According to these guidelines, circumstances in which comanagement would be appropriate include the following:

- The operating ophthalmologist and nonoperating practitioner provide postoperative care within an integrated health system such as the Veterans

Administration Health System or the Department of Defense in which both the operating ophthalmologist and nonoperating practitioner are employees of the parent entity and, as such, do not directly participate in Medicare comanagement. The protocol for comanagement or transfer of care emphasizes patient safety, and the timing of this transfer is based on postoperative stability and patient preference.

- Patient's inability to return to the operating ophthalmologist's office for follow-up care
  - ○ The patient is unable to travel to the ophthalmologist's office because of distance.
  - ○ There is a lack of availability of the person(s) or organization previously responsible for bringing the patient to the operating ophthalmologist's office.
- Operating ophthalmologist's unavailability
  - ○ The operating ophthalmologist will be unavailable to provide care (eg, travel, illness, or leave or surgery performed in an ophthalmologist shortage area).
- Patient's prerogative
  - ○ The patient requests comanagement or transfer of care to minimize cost of travel, loss of time spent traveling, or the patient's inconvenience and gives informed written consent to the comanagement arrangement or the transfer of care, and the operating ophthalmologist is familiar with the nonoperating practitioner and is confident that the practitioner has the adequate training, skills, and experience to accurately diagnose and treat the conditions that are likely to be presented as well as the willingness of the nonoperating practitioner to seek advice from operating ophthalmologists whenever necessary.
- Change in postoperative course
  - ○ The development of another illness or complication best handled by another qualified health care provider
  - ○ The development of an intercurrent disease

They went on to specify comanagement and transfer of care arrangements should be conducted using written patient-specific protocols to ensure the following criteria are met:

- The patient requests *and* makes an informed decision in writing to be seen by the nonoperating practitioner for postoperative care.
- The operating ophthalmologist determines that the operative eye is sufficiently stable for transfer of care or comanagement.

- The operating ophthalmologist determines that the transfer of care or co-management arrangement is clinically appropriate.
- The nonoperating practitioner is willing to accept the care of the patient.
- State law permits the nonoperating practitioner to provide postoperative care, and the nonoperating practitioner is otherwise qualified to do so.
- The operating ophthalmologist is familiar with the nonoperating practitioner and is confident that the practitioner has the adequate training, skills, and experience to accurately diagnose and treat the conditions that are likely to be presented as well as the willingness of the nonoperating practitioner to seek advice from operating ophthalmologists whenever necessary.
- There is no agreement or understanding between the operating ophthalmologist and a referring nonoperating practitioner to automatically send patients back to the nonoperating practitioner.
- The arrangement complies with all applicable federal and state laws and regulations, including the federal Anti-Kickback Statute, Stark Law, and state laws concerning fee splitting and patient brokering.[2]
- The operating ophthalmologist or an appropriately trained ophthalmologist is available upon request from either the patient or nonoperating practitioner to provide medically necessary care related to the surgical procedure directly or indirectly to the patient.
- Financial compensation to the nonoperating practitioner is consistent with the following principles:
  - The nonoperating practitioner's comanagement fees should be commensurate with the service(s) actually provided and should be separately billed by the nonoperating practitioner.
  - For Medicare/Medicaid patients, the comanagement arrangement should be consistent with all Medicare/Medicaid billing and coding rules and should not result in higher charges to Medicare/Medicaid than would occur without comanagement.
  - The patient should be informed of, and consent in writing to, any financial compensation to the nonoperating practitioner resulting from the comanagement arrangement and any additional fees that the nonoperating practitioner may charge beyond those covered by Medicare/Medicaid or other third-party payers.
  - For services that are not covered by Medicare/Medicaid, other fee structures may be appropriate, although they should also be commensurate

with the services provided, disclosed, and consented to in writing by the patient and otherwise comply with all applicable federal and state laws and regulations.

- Transfer of care or comanagement is documented in the medical record as required by carrier policy.
- All relevant clinical information is exchanged between the operating ophthalmologist and the nonoperating practitioner.

Recall the Stark Law prohibits physicians from making referrals for designated health services payable by Medicare if the physician or an immediate family member has a financial relationship with the entity to which the physician refers. Payments to physicians under a comanagement agreement constitute a financial relationship, which places them at risk of violation of the Stark Law. Stark Law exceptions are available to protect payments under a reasonable comanagement agreement. Exceptions require that the compensation paid by the surgeon to the physicians rendering postoperative care be set in advance, remain constant, not reflect volume or value of referrals, and reflect fair market value of the services provided. For example, a comanagement arrangement in which the doctor rendering postoperative care receives $1000 for a femtosecond laser–assisted phacoemulsification procedure would be over the fair market value.

STRUCTURING THE COMANAGEMENT AGREEMENT

Drafting a comanagement agreement between the surgeon and doctor(s) providing postoperative care is suggested. Within this document, the following elements should be included to comply with the various regulatory rules:

- Establishment of compensation in advance
- Agreement structured so as not to induce or reward physicians for increased referrals
- Adequate descriptions of services to be provided, including communication with the surgeon and when to return patients to the surgeon for care
- Support by an independent, third-party valuation to ensure that the listed compensation is appropriate
- Periodic reviews or audits to verify prohibited actions are not included
- Allowance of physicians to make independent decisions based on the patient's medical needs
- A limited duration of the agreement, typically 3 years

Furthermore, a consent for comanagement agreement[19] between the patient and surgeon is also required. This is typically signed while scheduling surgery. Ophthalmic Mutual Insurance Company states patients need to know which aspects of their care are delegated to a comanaging doctor and that they may contact the surgeon and return to him or her for care at any time. Ophthalmologists in Florida should use a specific Florida comanagement consent form[20] to meet the requirements of Florida state law.

CODE OF ETHICS

Most professional groups have published guidelines. Sections relating to marketing communications follow.

American Academy of Ophthalmology Code of Ethics

13. **Communications to the Public**. Communications to the public must be accurate. They must not convey false, untrue, deceptive, or misleading information through statements, testimonials, photographs, graphics or other means. They must not omit material information without which the communications would be deceptive. Communications must not appeal to an individual's anxiety in an excessive or unfair way; and they must not create unjustified expectations of results. If communications refer to benefits or other attributes of ophthalmic procedures that involve significant risks, realistic assessments of their safety and efficacy must also be included, as well as the availability of alternatives and, where necessary to avoid deception, descriptions and/or assessments of the benefits or other attributes of those alternatives. Communications must not misrepresent an ophthalmologist's credentials, training, experience or ability, and must not contain material claims of superiority that cannot be substantiated. If a communication results from payment by an ophthalmologist, this must be disclosed unless the nature, format or medium makes it apparent.[21]

Ethical marketing can improve your reputation and build your brand as well as loyal relationships. Unethical marketing can destroy your reputation, drive patients away, and result in legal problems.

American Academy of Optometry Code of Ethics, Section 5

SECTION 5

THE PROFESSIONAL STANDARDS OF MEMBERS OF THE ACADEMY REQUIRE THAT PUBLIC STATEMENTS, ANNOUNCEMENTS, AND PROMOTIONAL ACTIVITIES NOT BE DECEPTIVE, FRAUDULENT, OR MISLEADING.

Since individual patients want to know, and have a right to know, more about vision care (including optometry and visual science) their best interests are served by the proper dissemination of information within specific guidelines.

Members of the American Academy of Optometry, when participating in public education efforts:

5.1 Are enjoined to function with the patient's best interest in mind and to stress optometry's goal to provide excellence in vision care to all patients.

5.2 Will ensure that public information statements are based on scientific knowledge and fact.

5.3 Will not misuse Academy membership when dealing with the public or the media.

5.4 Must ensure that, when applicable, statements regarding eye care should follow the usual application of informed consent, noting alternative therapy, complications and efficacy of proposed treatment.

5.5 Shall not compensate nor give anything of value, including services, to a representative of the press, radio, television, or other communications media in anticipation of, or return for, professional publicity in a news item.

5.6 Should understand that the Academy is concerned that some optometrists may unintentionally mislead the public by using statements which can be misconstrued and that there may be a few who might attempt to attract patients through statements which are false and misleading. The Academy asserts that such statements are not in the public interest and constitute conduct unworthy of Academy members.[22]

American Optometric Association Social Media Recommendations

The AOA published recommendations for social networking and internet usage in November 2012. The AOA directed optometrists to uphold the ethical standards in the office when managing their online presence. The following recommendations were created to preserve the doctor-patient relationship, maintain privacy of patients, and protect information:

1. Interacting with past or current patients on social media platforms such as Instagram, Twitter, and Facebook is discouraged.

2. Discussing medical treatment with patients over social media should be done only after the identity of the patient is verified.

3. Discussion between colleagues should be done on secure networks on sites requiring registration. Passwords should be used to protect health information.

4. Protect patient privacy by avoiding the use of actual names or code names, pictures, or identifying information.

5. When writing online material, optometrists should disclose any financial conflicts of interest.

6. Be aware that your online statements may be reposted. Be sure information posted is factual.

7. Employee policy regarding internet use and social media should be created for each office.

8. Personal email should be different from the email address used professionally.

9. Professionalism online should be at the same level as expected within the office.[23]

REFERENCES

1. Wong S. They claimed what? 10 products with outrageous marketing claims. Published March 12, 2012. Accessed March 9, 2019. https://groups.google.com/g/opendebateforum/c/xUBkihtrHRY/m/UcV9shKtzIYJ?pli=1

2. Burnham T. Nutella maker may settle deceptive ad lawsuit for $3 million. *NPR*. Published April 26, 2012. Accessed August 6, 2020. https://www.npr.org/sections/thesalt/2012/04/26/151454929/nutella-maker-may-settle-deceptive-ad-lawsuit-for-3-million

3. Young S. Kellogg settles Rice Krispies false ad case. Published June 4, 2010. Accessed March 9, 2019. http://thechart.blogs.cnn.com/2010/06/04/kellogg-settles-rice-krispies-false-ad-case/

4. Sweney M. Twiggy's Olay ad banned over airbrushing. *The Guardian*. Published December 16, 2009. Accessed August 6, 2020. https://www.theguardian.com/media/2009/dec/16/twiggys-olay-ad-banned-airbrushing

5. US Food and Drug Administration. Misleadingly labeled e-liquids that appeal to youth. Updated July 20, 2020. Accessed August 6, 2020. https://www.fda.gov/TobaccoProducts/NewsEvents/ucm605729.htm

6. Heilpern W. 18 False advertising scandals that cost some brands millions. Business Insider. Published March 31, 2016. Accessed August 6, 2020. https://www.businessinsider.com/false-advertising-scandals-2016-3#activia-yogurt-said-it-had-special-bacterial-ingredients-2

7. Wal-Mart settles false advertising case. Corporate Crime Reporter. Published September 16, 2014. Accessed August 6, 2020. https://www.corporatecrimereporter.com/news/200/wal-mart-settles-false-advertising-case/

8. FDA warns maker of Latisse about misleading claims. Consumer Reports News. Published September 17, 2009. Accessed March 9, 2019. https://www.consumerreports.org/cro/news/2009/09/fda-warns-maker-of-latisse-about-misleading-claims/index.htm

9. Ruiz R. Ten misleading drug ads. Forbes.com. Published February 2, 2019. Accessed March 5, 2019. https://www.forbes.com/2010/02/02/drug-advertising-lipitor-lifestyle-health-pharmaceuticals-safety_slide.html#599b246a2398

10. Goldblatt D, Naumann R. Justin Timberlake accused of deceiving consumers in class action lawsuit over Bai Brands beverages. The Blast. Published May 3, 2018. Accessed March 10, 2019. https://theblast.com/justin-timberlake-bai-brands-beverages-lawsuit/

11. Minato C. 10 recent racist ads that companies wish you could forget. Business Insider. Published June 7, 2012. Accessed August 6, 2020. https://www.businessinsider.com/the-10-most-racist-ads-of-the-modern-era-2012-6#intel-released-an-ad-they-knew-was-racist-7

12. Martins AT. 10 examples of unethical marketing practices that ruin reputation. Profitable Venture Magazine LLC. Accessed August 7, 2020. https://www.profitableventure.com/examples-unethical-marketing-practices/

13. Dobkowski M. 10 steps to help your ophthalmology practice avoid SEO malpractice. Published January 5, 2009. Accessed March 5, 2019. http://www.interactiverefractive.com/10-steps-to-help-your-ophthalmology-practice-avoid-seo-malpractice/

14. Brendel AM. Navigating the comanagement waters: it can be treacherous, so don't go it alone. Ophthalmology Management. Published March 1, 2018. Accessed March 4, 2019. https://www.ophthalmologymanagement.com/issues/2018/march-2018/navigating-the-co-management-waters

15. Medicare and State Health Care Programs: Fraud and Abuse; Clarification of the Initial OIG Safe Harbor Provisions and Establishment of Additional Safe Harbor Provisions Under the Anti-Kickback Statute. *Fed Regist.* 1999;64(223):63518,63548-63549. 42 CFR 1001.

16. American Optometric Association. Optometric postoperative care. Published April 27, 2000. Accessed August 7, 2020. https://www.aoa.org/Documents/about/06b_Other_AOA_Postoperative_Care_Position_Paper.pdf

17. Morris L. OIG advisory opinion no. 11-14. Department of Health and Human Services: Office of Inspector General. Published October 7, 2011. Accessed August 7, 2020. https://oig.hhs.gov/fraud/docs/advisoryopinions/2011/AdvOpn11-14.pdf

18. American Academy of Ophthalmology. Comprehensive guidelines for the co-management of ophthalmic postoperative care. Published September 7, 2016. Accessed August 7, 2020. https://www.aao.org/ethics-detail/guidelines-comanagement-postoperative-care#one

19. Ophthalmic Mutual Insurance Company: A Risk Retention Group. Sample informed consent document. Accessed August 7, 2020. https://www.omic.com/wp-content/uploads/2018/07/Consent-for-comanagement-of-surgical-patients.docx

20. Ophthalmic Mutual Insurance Company: A Risk Retention Group. Florida co-management law mandates new informed consent process. Updated 2020. Accessed August 7, 2020. https://www.omic.com/tips/alert-change-to-florida-co-management-law-mandates-new-informed-consent-requirements/

21. American Academy of Ophthalmology. Code of ethics. Published January 1, 2020. Accessed August 7, 2020. https://www.aao.org/ethics-detail/code-of-ethics#public

22. American Academy of Optometry. Fellowship standards. Accessed August 7, 2020. https://www.aaopt.org/membership/member-resources/fellowship-standards

23. Carman C, Totten D. Social media recommendations. American Optometric Association. Published November 2012. Accessed August 25, 2020. https://www.aoa.org/about-the-aoa/ethics-and-values?sso=y

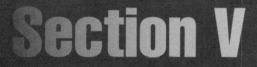

Section V

Disruptive Technologies and Future Directions

16

Disruptive Technologies and Trends That Will Impact Marketing

Kane Harrison

In *The Innovator's Dilemma: When New Technologies Cause Great Firms to Fail*, Clayton Christensen[1] wrote that disruption occurs when a technology's performance surpasses customer needs. When that happens, the basis of competition changes, and a new technology arrives that outperforms the incumbent on some other parameter. He further categorizes new technology as *sustaining* or *disruptive*.[1] Sustaining technology relies on incremental improvements to an established technology. Disruptive technology is new, lacks refinement, and may suffer performance problems initially. It appeals to a limited audience and may not have a proven practical application upon launch.

The automobile was once a disruptive technology. When early adapters to automobiles were driving on dirt roads in the United States, overtaking horse-drawn carts with newfound egos from increased social status, they could not have imagined what was about to unfurl. Internationally, drivers fell in love with the automobile as a predominant form of transportation, and US consumers accumulated over $1.1 trillion in auto debt.[2] Despite banner growth, a new

Wang M, ed. *Grow Your Eye Care Practice:*
High-Impact Pearls From the Marketing Experts (pp 149-155).
© 2021 Taylor & Francis Group.

trend emerged—the number of people getting a driver's license has steadily declined.[3] Although more and more teens and people in their 20s are foregoing driver's licenses, the most recent trend holds true for pretty much all age groups according to the University of Michigan researchers.[3]

In a new report examining changes in driver licensure in the United States from 1983 to 2014, Michael Sivak and Brandon Schoettle of the University of Michigan Transportation Research Institute found a continuous decrease in the percentage of those under 45 years of age with a license.[3] Even the proportion of Americans 45 to 69 years of age with driver's licenses has declined overall since 2008, following a 25-year rise.

This shift in the car-buying environment led to alternative transportation solutions such as Uber and Lyft. The ripple effects of auto industry disruption can be felt across insurance, parts suppliers, fuel companies, and any industry adjacent to transportation.

Examples of disruptive technology within the health care field include artificial intelligence, immunomodulation treatments, liquid biopsy, gene therapy, and 3-dimensional printing of body parts. Bionic eye and brain implants are currently under development.[4] Within eye care, we have several examples of disruptive technology that are now considered standard of care. Imagine what the inventor of the ophthalmoscope would say if he saw retinal optimal coherence tomography or full-field retinal photography. Visual field–testing using computer algorithms, contact tonometry without anesthetic, and excimer and femtosecond laser treatments are used daily in practice.

The internet has affected eye care as well. Online contact lens and spectacle purchases are now mainstream. Online contact lens purchases have been slowly creeping upward from 17.5% in 2013 to about 19% in 2016.[5] Brands sold exclusively via the internet rather than by an eye doctor have emerged. Online eye exams have emerged as well, with Visibly (formerly Opternative) continuing to fight the battle for the ability to prescribe glasses using only online testing. Eight million pairs of prescription eyeglasses were sold online in 2017. This represented only 4.2% of the total prescription eyeglass market in the United States.[6]

Warby Parker, a now infamous American eyewear disrupter, began operating online exclusively in 2010. In 2018, Vox.com reported that on March 14, 2018, Warby Parker raised $75 million in Series E funding, making its total funding about $300 million.[7] As of the article's release, the new funding values the New York City–based company at a pre–initial public offering valuation of $1.75 billion. Warby Parker accomplished this in 10 years, unlike the 100 years the automobile trend required.

DISRUPTIVE TECHNOLOGY

Potential patients are displaying an intense desire for customized engagements and content across channels, particularly on mobile devices. As a result, patient experience, patient retention and growth, and patient analytics will be the most vital areas to support marketing outcomes in the foreseeable future. The eye care companies, and more specifically the service providers, that are driven by technological advancements specific to customer acquisition will be more successful.

It is not a secret that eye care marketers and business owners are struggling to develop personalized patient experiences across the buying journey. They are under tremendous pressure to find the right tools to achieve results-based outcomes and track patient-centric trends. Patient expectations for personalized interaction are higher than ever. Business leaders are more commonly requiring transparency in marketing to monitor their return on investment.

The classic 4 Ps in marketing are price, product, promotion, and place. These have been the foothold for those marketing eye care over the years, but we have moved well beyond the local newspaper, billboards, and TV. Although these can be a part of your overall strategy, emerging technology now affects all 4 Ps across the entire marketing ecosystem. With a mixture of programmatic advertising including automated buying and selling of online advertising, conversational bots, and dynamic pricing models executed by personal virtual agents, the competition for potential patients' attention is competitive.

To lead a technology-driven strategy and innovate, we must be willing to explore future scenarios, distinguish improvements, prepare for disruptions, and take an outside-in view. Only those who can navigate the changing environment while identifying and prioritizing new technologies will succeed.

Disruptive Trends

Patients are becoming numb to brand interactions that are not authentic, such as $299 LASIK advertisements, or relevant, such as advertising solutions for presbyopia to a young myopic demographic. They want the brands they respect to demonstrate a thorough understanding of their preferences, offer personalized interactions, and make a social impact. Patients are redefining brand value on their terms, demanding greater convenience and relevance from each engagement across their devices.

Trust and Values

According to Gartner Iconoculture data, consumer trust and values are undergoing a fundamental shift.[8] Ninety-three percent of consumers trust locally owned businesses, whereas only 41% trust corporate America. Trust is now intimate, small, and local. Meanwhile, serenity is the fastest rising value for consumers polled by Iconoculture. This refers to consumers seeking calm peaceful surroundings and situations. This is followed by security and inclusion. Marketers who understand these shifting values and beliefs will be better positioned to compete in the dynamic eye care landscape.

Trends That Shape Your Environment

Political, economic, and cultural polarization have a profound effect on marketers' ability to be successful. More often than not your patients obtain information about their environment through the same channel you are marketing through. If a patient is viewing content via a channel that has a particular bias that does not align with the views of the patient, the patient can feel an unwarranted bias toward your content if displayed in the same environment. We must understand these dynamics to compete effectively. Consumers are more divided today compared with a generation ago, and the polarization effect is not confined to politics. There is a widening economic gap in the United States. In the current environment, a brand story extends beyond the carefully crafted messages shaped by an organization. Today's patients are self-educators, and anything that is knowable about a brand is now part of your brand story.

Content Expectations

Ninety percent of brands practice at least one form of marketing personalization, but the content will be the bottleneck, and improper use of content will cause failure. Most marketers fail to realize that even with extensive patient data, they do not have adequate content to deliver what potential patients expect. Marketing organizations that reimagine the creative brief and segment their content into atoms for targeting will be better equipped to capitalize on personalized experiences by uniting customer data with relevant content.

Voice-Driven Search Queries

At the 2019 American Society of Cataract and Refractive Surgery meeting in San Diego, California, the predominant question regarding disruptive trends was about conversation agents, such as Alexa (in reference to Amazon's Alexa) and personal assistants such as Google. Adopter brands that redesign their websites to support visual and voice search will increase digital traffic, digital-driven revenue, and market share. Voice-driven search queries are on track to become the dominant search mode for mobile users.

As voice search grows, it will completely upend tried-and-true practices around paid search and organic content strategy. In the very near future, conversational agents like Amazon's Alexa will begin to meditate more transactions with patients. It is important to understand the following 2 things about Alexa:

1. Alexa is a conversational agent, a software program that chats with humans through face-to-face conversation and uses anthropomorphic (ie, having human characteristics) techniques.

2. Amazon is not Google. They are competing companies with different motivations.

Optimize Your Website for Voice Assistants

These are 5 technical tune-ups to optimize your website to rank in Alexa's search. The Alexa search engine optimization (SEO) audit tool (available at https://try.alexa.com/marketing-stack/seo-audit-tool) may assist with this adaptation. There are a lot of small, technical things you must do to make sure that it is as easy as possible for search engines to find and understand your site's content. Although simple, these elements can have a big effect on your site's visibility. There are 4 basic SEO elements on a site:

1. The title tag is the blue link displayed in search results, on external websites, and in browser tabs. Generally, it defines the title of a document and is important for social sharing and for SEO. It is best practice to keep the title tag under 65 characters, so it will fit in the search engine results display.

2. The meta description is the text that is included underneath your title tag. It is a concise description (approximately 155 characters) of the page's content and is the first interaction a prospective visitor has with your site. Think of the meta description as the elevator pitch for your web page or website. It serves as a compelling description that you hope will entice the visitor to click through.

3. The H1 tag tells crawlers/bots what to expect on a page. There is only one H1 tag per page, and it should be similar to the page title tag. If the H1 tag

is the question your user might be searching for, the associated content is the answer. Optimizing information based on users' questions and adding appropriately placed keywords will reward in improved search engine placement.

4. Alt tags are the behind-the-scenes descriptions of content, like images, on your website. They describe an image when it is unable to be seen, and search engines use them to decipher the image or give context to the corresponding content. Alt tags should use concise, descriptive, keyword-relevant text. This is important so search engines can interpret them properly but also because visually impaired visitors using screen readers will hear alt text when visiting a website.

Duplicate Content

If not handled properly, duplicate content can be damaging to your SEO. Multiple copies of content can dilute the authority of your page, and because Google usually filters out duplicate content from the search results, it is possible for the wrong version of a page to be displayed as a search result. In other words, search engines are forced to decide which version of the duplicate content is most relevant to searches.

Broken Links

Broken links can be a huge detriment to your users' experience, resulting in lost conversions and sales. For search engines, a broken link is a signal of a poor-quality site, which may negatively affect ranks. Broken links can be caused by renaming or moving a web page and failing to change internal links, linking to content that has been moved or deleted, or linking to a third-party page that changed the URL or changed the page. Even if your own site has not changed, the links or pages on other sites may no longer work. A regular site audit will check both your internal and external links to make sure you are not confusing your visitors or search engine crawlers with broken links.

HTML Tags and Certified Metrics

You make business decisions based on the data from your on-site analytics tags. It is important to make sure that the code for each of your web analytics products (eg, Alexa Certified Metrics, Google Analytics, Facebook Pixels) are all properly added so you can be sure all of your site's traffic is counted and tracked. Regular site audits will make sure that as you add new content to your site, all pages are covered and your on-site analytics are as accurate as possible.

Site Performance

Your website's performance affects both your visitors' experience and your search engine rankings. A study from the Alexa Blog (https://blog.alexa.com) reports that 47% of people expect a web page to load in 2 seconds or less.[9] With just seconds to make an impression on visitors, page load time is the last thing you want to stand between you and conversions. In terms of SEO, Google has reported in the Webmaster Central Blog[10] that page speed is one element factored into page rank algorithms.

Disruptive technology will continue to shift health care, and it is imperative we are responsive to these trends.

REFERENCES

1. Christensen CM. *The Innovator's Dilemma: When New Technologies Cause Great Firms to Fail.* Harvard Business School Press Boston; 1997:10-11.

2. Fontinelle A. American debt: auto loan balances total $1.2 trillion in 2020. Accessed August 14, 2019. https://www.investopedia.com/personal-finance/american-debt-auto-loan-debt/

3. University of Michigan Transportation Research Institute. More Americans of all ages spurning driver's licenses. Published January 20, 2016. Accessed August 7, 2020. http://www.umtri.umich.edu/what-were-doing/news/more-americans-all-ages-spurning-drivers-licenses

4. The Medical Futurist. The future of vision and eye care. Published October 26, 2017. Accessed August 7, 2020. https://medicalfuturist.com/future-of-vision-and-eye-care

5. Shahbandeh M. Contact lenses in the U.S. - statistics & facts. Published July 13, 2018. Accessed June 23, 2019. https://www.statista.com/topics/4570/contact-lenses-in-the-us/

6. Kestenbaum R. Buying glasses online is becoming the norm—but growth will explode once eye exams go digital. Published April 24, 2018. Accessed June 23, 2019. https://www.forbes.com/sites/richardkestenbaum/2018/04/24/online-eyeglasses-has-explosive-growth-ahead-of-it/#55f5397527c8

7. Del Rey J. Warby Parker is valued at $1.75 billion after a pre-IPO investment of $75 million. Published March 14, 2018. Accessed August 14, 2019. https://www.vox.com/2018/3/14/17115230/warby-parker-75-million-funding-t-rowe-price-ipo

8. McCall T. Gartner says pressure is on marketers to think big, execute smart and deliver growth. Gartner. Published May 15, 2018. Accessed August 25, 2020. https://www.gartner.com/en/newsroom/press-releases/2018-05-15-gartner-says-pressure-is-on-marketers-to-think-big-execute-smart-and-deliver-growth

9. Work S. How loading time affects your bottom line. NeilPatel.com. Accessed August 7, 2020. https://neilpatel.com/blog/loading-time/

10. Singhal A, Cutts M. Using site speed in web search ranking. Google Webmaster Central Blog. Published April 9, 2010. Accessed August 25, 2020. https://webmasters.googleblog.com/.

17

Future Marketing Trends

John Mickner, BA; Michael Weiss, BS, MBA; Robbie W. Grayson III, BA;
Joshua Frenkel, MD, MPH; Arun C. Gulani, MD, MS; and Ming Wang, MD, PhD

When talking about the future of marketing with doctors, they tend to focus on the patient experience and using word-of-mouth marketing on social media. The future has come full circle to "word of mouth." The medium has changed from word of mouth on street corners and coffee shops to online social media. The speed of transmission over an Internet that never "closes" enables immediate sharing of patient experiences. Practitioners must be mindful that this applies to both patients reporting gratifications and annoyances. Planning marketing strategies should encompass this expansive reach and speed of execution.[1]

John Mickner and other authors of this text who specialize in marketing feel it is more complicated. Given their vast understanding of marketing and advertising, this is expected. Small businesses lack the resources to compete with franchises and large corporate chains. For this reason, small practices often rely on a combination of retaining current customers and word-of-mouth marketing. In the past, these strategies were adequate to keep the business

Wang M, ed. *Grow Your Eye Care Practice:*
High-Impact Pearls From the Marketing Experts (pp 157-161).
© 2021 Taylor & Francis Group.

afloat or even prosper. Today, additional marketing methods must be added to be competitive. Strategies of customer retention and word-of-mouth marketing worked well when you were the only game in town but are less effective with competition nearby. With today's mergers and acquisitions, franchising opportunities, and organic expansion by large corporations, competition has exponentially increased. Lack of marketing plans in a changing competitive landscape negatively affects small business growth.

Future trends that practitioners should consider include the following:

- Increasing patient expectations: As mobility and online interactions continue, increasing expectations for complete online interaction with the office are likely. This includes both the desktop and mobile experience for the patient. As widespread usage of third-party software tools improve, the patient will expect his or her interactive experiences to continue to improve. This may result in less personal interaction and more communication via SMS and email. This is a tricky area for medical professionals given Health Insurance Portability and Accountability Act laws. It is not as simple as using FaceTime (Apple), texting a patient, or sending an email. Health Insurance Portability and Accountability Act–compliant secure messaging applications are required and are currently available using third-party software.

- Data security and privacy: Data security and privacy will play an increased role in the future of marketing because the risks of data breach of patient communications are both real and expensive.

- Better data analysis for making decisions: Better population data and collection methods will become available, enabling practitioners to make more even informed marketing decisions. Subpopulations of prospective patients based on desired traits will be easier to identify and communicate with.

- Increasing focus on quality vs quantity: As artificial intelligence (AI) and search engines improve, websites that do not meet patient experience requirements or contain less reputable content will fall in ranking. The search engine optimization tricks that work now will be less effective in the future.

- Unforeseen disruptions: As mobile devices and tablets disrupted how we interact with the internet and communicate, disruptions lie ahead that will require doctors to adapt their strategies. If self-driving cars become a reality, it will change how people spend their time driving. As tablets, smartphones, and computers evolve, people may change their expectations and usage habits. New legislation will also develop, and practitioners must incorporate this as well.

Emerging technologies and trends that will specifically affect how practitioners market include many of the following:

- Atomic content: Atomic content structure allows users to select the information they need without forcing them to sort through information they do not want. Users can easily find the "atom" of content they need. Atomic content represents the building blocks of more advanced and comprehensive forms of personalization and makes it easier to determine (through analytics) what content is used more often. This next wave of personalization will customize multiple dimensions of a consumer's experience based on demographic, psychographic, and behavioral data.

- Programmatic placement: Programmatic placement is buying digital advertising space automatically, with computers using data to decide which ads to buy and how much to pay for them. Programmatic placement puts brands everywhere. Programmatic advertising has been growing for almost a decade and continues its steady march beyond the internet into native mobile formats, television, radio, and out-of-home media.

- Shopping chatbots: A new generation of shopping chatbots go beyond immediately answering simple queries. A computer program automatically searches the internet for particular products or services, compares their prices, and often gives customers' opinions of their quality. These shopping chatbots are immune to marketing tactics that draw on human emotion.

- Dynamic pricing: Dynamic pricing, also referred to as *surge pricing, demand pricing,* or *time-based pricing,* is a pricing strategy in which businesses set flexible prices for products or services based on current market demands. Most of us have seen this style of pricing with companies like Uber. Dynamic pricing algorithms are now used across large and small enterprises. Pricing is an important and increasingly dynamic element of marketing strategy for nonmedical businesses. This may be less of an issue for medical services.

- Smart contracts: Smart contracts can be fully executed in computer code without the requirement of physical documentation, and they enable autonomous negotiation among smart agents of buyers and sellers. The transactions between payers/providers and patients/providers will become more efficient. Smart contracts will create new virtual marketplaces and change how eye care services are sought and presented to consumers.

- The sharing economy: The sharing economy already disrupts our notion of sales and ownership. Many eye care providers share a surgery center rather than own one for example. Every industry needs to look ahead and see how and where sharing dynamics will have an effect and how this may change their basic value proposition.

- Anthropomorphic voice of things and internet of things: Anthropomorphic (ie, having human characteristics) voice of things and internet of things technologies are becoming ingrained in our culture. Anthropomorphic techniques that use human language and symbolism and devices such as virtual assistants and chatbots can promote natural interaction, trust, learning, and empathy between AI software/models and humans. Medical providers must tread lightly in this arena because a strong anthropomorphic approach is not always best. In sensitive situations such as providing medical advice to a user, overly anthropomorphic approaches could make patients uncomfortable and prevent them from disclosing essential information.

- Multitouch attribution (MTA): MTA is a way to allocate credit toward marketing touch points that preceded a conversion within a patient's journey. When you couple MTA with atomic content, you have the power to analyze each marketing touch point definitively. Marketers using MTA find they can better allocate their budgets to those touch points that work best for any one particular outcome.

- Cross-device identification: Cross-device identification can match a smartphone, laptop, tablet, smart watch, smart TV, or any connected device to a specific individual and track how consumers use these devices to navigate between websites, social channels, and public portals. Sophisticated ad targeting, personalization, and measurement capabilities allow the delivery of a consistent content experience for potential and existing patients across user channels.

- Predictive analytics: Predictive analytics is a variant of machine learning that anticipates future behaviors and estimates unknown outcomes. Marketing leaders explore its potential for churn management, cross-selling, propensity to purchase, multichannel campaign management, and customer lifetime value prediction as well as new applications to improve business decision making.

- AI: AI has the potential to revolutionize patient interactions over the next decade by enabling conversational experiences, real-time personalization, and content generation. This may be used for diagnosis and treatment as algorithms are developed as well as how patients interact with practice websites.

- Customer data platforms: A customer data platform is a type of packaged software that creates a persistent, unified customer database that is accessible to other systems. Data are pulled from multiple sources, cleaned, and combined to create a single customer profile. These structured data are then made available to other marketing systems. Customer data platforms have the potential to transform how you deliver consistent, targeted, and relevant patient experiences.

Overall, marketing will become a technology hub. General marketing skills taught in professional schools often used in the past will become less important. Practitioners need to invest in understanding how to use newer technologies before they become a realized commodity. The smarter technology becomes, the less personal interactions between doctor and patient will occur.

Reference

1. Roshni M. Dr. Arun Gulani. *Roshni Magazine.* Published August 16, 2009. Accessed August 26, 2020. https://roshnimagazine.wordpress.com/2009/08/16/dr-arun-gulani/

Financial Disclosures

Dr. Joshua Frenkel has no financial or proprietary interest in the materials presented herein.

Robbie W. Grayson III has no financial or proprietary interest in the materials presented herein.

Dr. Arun C. Gulani is a consultant to Biotissue, Oculus, CorneaGen, and Marco.

Kane Harrison has no financial or proprietary interest in the materials presented herein.

James E. Looper Jr has no financial or proprietary interest in the materials presented herein.

Shareef Mahdavi has no financial or proprietary interest in the materials presented herein.

Catherine Maley has no financial or proprietary interest in the materials presented herein.

Michael Malley has no financial or proprietary interest in the materials presented herein.

John Mickner has no financial or proprietary interest in the materials presented herein.

Dr. Karl Stonecipher has no financial or proprietary interest in the materials presented herein.

Dr. Tracy Schroeder Swartz has no financial or proprietary interest in the materials presented herein.

Dr. Ming Wang has no financial or proprietary interest in the materials presented herein.

Michael Weiss is CEO and co-founder of MedForward, Inc.

Jeremy Westby has no financial or proprietary interest in the materials presented herein.

Index

Printed in the United States
by Baker & Taylor Publisher Services

Printed in the United States
by Baker & Taylor Publisher Services